HERBALISM FOR BEGINNERS

A Beginners Guide to Herbal Remedies and Medicine. Discover the Common Herbs and Spices You Can Grow At Home.

Arin Gladstar

The data, facts and description of events forthwith shall be considered as accurate unless the work is deemed to be a work of fiction. In any event, the Publisher is exempt of responsibility for any use of the information contained in the present work on the part of the user. The author and Publisher may not be deemed liable, under any circumstances, for the events resulting from the observance of the advice, tips, techniques and any other contents presented herein.

Given the informational and entertainment nature of the content presented in this work, there is no guarantee as to the quality and validity of the information. As such, the contents of this work are deemed as universal. No use of copyrighted material is used in this work. Any references to other trademarks are done so under fair use and by no means represent an endorsement of such trademarks or their holder.

DISCLAIMER

The content of this book is not intended to be a substitute for professional medical advice, diagnosis, or treatment. The reader should always seek the advice of his/her physician or other qualified health provider with any questions you may have regarding a medical condition, including his/her diet.

Table of Contents

Chapter 1: The Wonderful World of Herbalism

For thousands of years, people from all cultures have been using plants for their medicinal properties. Long before the modern medicines that we are familiar with, which only emerged in the 20th century, families would often create their own remedies from plants grown in their gardens or 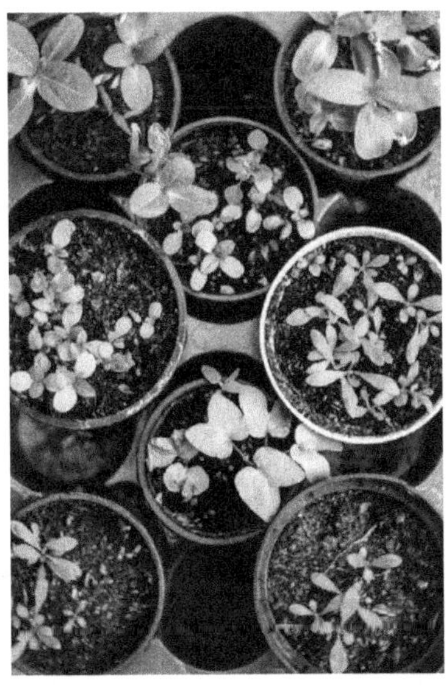 foraged in the wild, and would consult local herbalists for advice on the correct preparations and doses. In fact, many of our modern pharmaceuticals are based on herbal preparations that have been used throughout history.

Unfortunately, today many people are not aware of the healing properties of plants and how they can be used. Although certain herbal preparations, like tea, can be widely found, not many people can identify why we drink tea from peppermint leaves, or what health benefits a tea from this particular herb may have.

Slowly, modern people are starting to rediscover the herbs that our ancestors were so familiar with and becoming familiar again with their healing properties and the important part that they can play in our lives today. If you are curious about how you can boost your immune system, relieve the pain of arthritis, and calm eczema right from your garden, then this book is for you.

Herbalism is the practice of using preparations from plants to treat common ailments, alleviate their symptoms, and even preventing the development of chronic conditions. There is also a sort of satisfaction in knowing where your remedies come from and taking control of your own wellness from growing the herbs through to preparing the herbal remedies. It is appealing to think that all of the medicines that are going into or onto your family's bodies have been created by your own knowledge of herbs.

In this book, *Easy Herbalism,* we will introduce you to 16 of the most common medicinal herbs that have been used for hundreds of years. We will discuss how to identify these herbs in the wild, talk about how they were used by our ancestors, and explain how to create medicinal preparations that can be used in the herbal first aid kit, including when and how to use them. Of the herbs that are listed in this book, you have probably heard of all of them before, others you might not be as familiar with. You may even have some of these herbs growing in your yard as weeds right now and not even know it.

Once you have become more familiar with the herbs listed in this book and have tried out some of the recipes included for creating your own herbal teas, oils, salves, tinctures, poultices, and more, you will find yourself reaching for these remedies more often, and increasing your overall wellness by incorporating them into your daily life. There are many recipes and suggestions included in this book, but once you have a grasp of the properties of each herb, you will feel comfortable creating your own blends based on what you have on hand and what properties you are looking to utilize.

There is so much to learn about herbs and what they can do for us. The herbs and recipes in this book are a great way to get started, but they are only the tip of the iceberg. Herbalism is more about acquiring knowledge and using this knowledge with some intuition to create the best preparations and mixtures for your needs.

Chapter 2: Benefits of Common Herbs

Not all herbs have the same benefits, and there are quite a few different ways that herbal preparations can act on the body. Before we learn more about the individual herbs, their properties, and how to create herbal medicines, it is important to understand how medications can work on the body. In this way, it will be possible to match the symptoms with the herbs that are needed for the specific issue.

It is important to note that most herbs will have several of the properties listed below, and there may be more than one herb that can work on an issue in the body. If we can understand how they work, then it will be possible to substitute different herbs when needed due to supply or taste. For example, two of the herbs that we will discuss, aloe vera and calendula, both work well when used on sunburn, but choosing which herb to use may depend somewhat on the other properties of the herb.

ANTIBACTERIAL – Anything that kills bacteria or stops the growth of bacteria in the body.
ANTIDIABETIC – A substance that helps to control the level of glucose (sugar) in the body.

ANTIFUNGAL – A drug that fights fungal infections, usually on the skin, scalp, or nails.

ANTIINFLAMMATORY – Something that reduces inflammation or swelling, which often also helps to reduce pain.

ANTIOXIDANT – Fights free radicals in the body. If free radical levels become too high, they can be linked to diseases such as diabetes, heart disease, and some cancers.

ANTIPROLIFERATIVE – Inhibits the growth of cells.

ANTIPRURITIC – Relieves itching caused by insect bites, sunburns, allergic reactions, eczema, psoriasis, and other causes.

ANTISEPTIC – An agent that prevents the growth of microorganisms that can cause disease by either limiting their activity or by destroying them.

ANTISPASMODIC – Relieves or suppresses involuntary muscle spasms.

ANTIULCERATIVE – Medications that block acid production, acid secretion, and prevent the formulation and healing of ulcers.

ANXIOLYTIC – Used to treat the symptoms of anxiety or stress, has a calming effect.

APHRODISIAC – An agent that can increase sexual desire.

ASTRINGENT – A substance that shrinks or constricts body tissues. Can reduce inflammation topically (on the skin).

CARMINATIVE – Any agent that has the ability to prevent or relieves gas and griping.

DECONGESTANT – Something that is used to relieve congestion, specifically of the nasal passages.

DEMULCENT – An agent that relieves irritation of mucous membranes by forming a protective film.

DIAPHORETIC – An agent that causes or encourages sweating.

DIGESTIVE – Used for its effect on the gastrointestinal system. Aids in gastrointestinal mobility, the breakdown of food, or the reduction of indigestion.

DIURETIC – A substance that increases the removal of water and salt from the body by increasing the as urine.

EMOLLIENT – An agent that softens the skin or moisturizes.

EXPECTORANT – Increase bronchial secretions and increase mucus flow so that they can be removed more easily through coughing.

GALACTAGOGUE – An agent that increases the production of milk.

LAXATIVE – Anything that stimulates or causes the evacuation of the bowels and reduction of constipation.

MUCOLYTIC – An agent that thins mucus. This makes the mucus easier to cough up because it is less sticky. Generally, these agents are used to treat respiratory conditions.

MUSCLE RELAXANT – An agent that is used to relieve the symptoms of muscle spasms and can relax muscles that have been overworked.

NERVINE – An agent that can calm nervous tension, nourish the nervous system, and can act as a sedative to the nervous system.

SEDATIVE – An agent that has the ability to promote a calm mood, or to induce sleep.

In addition to the different ways that the herbs can act on the body, there are different ways that the herbs can be applied to the body. With herbal medications, there are two main routes:

INGESTED – Medication taken orally, either as food, a pill, syrup, or tea, etc.

TOPICAL – Medication applied directly to the skin as a salve, compress, etc.

Chapter 3: Healthy and Effective Herbs and What We Know About Them

To get you started off with using herbs, there are a few common plants that are endlessly useful in your herbal first aid kit, and some of them may even be growing in your garden already. This book will focus on the following 16 herbs:

- Aloe Vera (Aloe Vera)
- Burdock (Arctium minus)
- Calendula (Calendula officinalis)
- Chickweed (Stellaria media)
- Dandelion (Taraxacum officinale)
- Echinacea (Echinacea purpurea)
- Elderflower (Sambucus nigra)
- Marshmallow (Althaea officinalis)
- Mullein (Verbascum Thapsus)
- Nettle (Urtica dioica)
- Oats (Avena sativa)
- Peppermint (Mentha piperita)
- Plantain (Plantago major)
- Red Clover (Trifolium pretense)
- Valerian (Valeriana officinalis)
- Yarrow (Achillea millefolium)

From this small group of herbs, it is possible to soothe burns, calm insect bites and allergic reactions, reduce fever, ease sore muscles, and help with many other common ailments.

After the discussion of the herbs and how they can help, we will discuss the different ways to prepare these herbs for use. Not every herb can be prepared the same way, and it is important to understand the properties of each herb so that their medicinal benefits may be maximized, and any potential contraindications are minimized.

There are many ways to use medicinal herbs, and we will outline and give recipes for some of the more common ways to prepare medicinal herbal preparations, including:

- Teas – infusions and decoctions of fresh or dried herbs.
- Syrups – herbs cooked into a sweet syrup with sugar or honey
- Oils – oils that are infused with herbs
- Salves – preparations made with herbs, oil, and beeswax used for topical purposes
- Tinctures – herbal infusion in alcohol
- Pills – a herbal paste made into pills, or powdered herbs added to gelatin capsules
- Poultices – herbs applied directly to the skin

- Compresses – herbal infusions applied to the skin

Each of these will be discussed, and by the end of this book, you will be confident in using your new herbal medicine knowledge.

Finally, we will touch on your herbal medicine cabinet, and give some ideas and recipes to include in your herbal first aid kit.

Aloe Vera (Aloe Vera)

Properties: Antipruritic, Digestive, Laxative, Skincare.

Common Uses: Digestive, Skin irritations (especially burns), Skincare.

Common Preparations: Salve, Directly on skin, Juice

Contraindications: Caution should be used when taking the gel orally. There is a chance that ingesting Aloe vera could cause abnormal heart rhythm or kidney problems in those with pre-existing heart or kidney issues. It may also lower blood sugar levels in diabetics. Ingestion may also negatively interact with prescription drugs used to treat clots, diabetes, heart disease, potassium-lowering agents, and diuretics. Topically, there is a rare potential for an allergic reaction or contact dermatitis. Do not take internally if pregnant.

Plant parts used: Gel from inside leaves.

Possible Side Effects

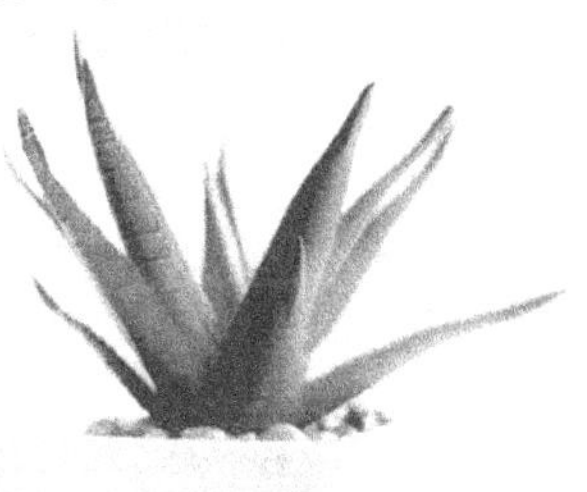

When harvesting the gel from an aloe vera plant,

especially for internal use, be sure to use only the white/clear gel inside the leaf and none of the leaf pulp or any yellow liquid latex from inside the leaf, which can be toxic or irritating to those with a latex allergy.

Plant Identification

Aloe vera is commonly grown as a houseplant, though it can be grown outdoors in warmer climates. It is a succulent with thick, dark green leaves growing directly from the ground, and is actually related to lilies and asparagus. When the leaves are cut, they are full of a gel-like substance, which is the useable part of the plant. The plant will typically have between 15-30 leaves, and each one will grow up to 12 inches long, and 3-4 inches wide.

An aloe vera plant will produce a spiky yellow cone-shaped flower when it reaches about 4 years of age. However, it is possible that indoor aloe vera plants will flower less frequently or not at all. The blooms appear in early spring and can last through the summer.

To harvest the gel, cut a leaf from the aloe plant, cutting close to the base of the plant, and leave the leaf to sit for about an hour. Wash and dry the leaf, and fillet by cutting up the two sides. Scrape off the white or clear gel with a spoon or knife, ensuring that none of the rind or yellow liquid is included.

The gel can be stored in the refrigerator for future use and used as-is or added to a salve, juice, or another recipe.

Historical Uses

The gel from the Aloe vera plant has been used medicinally for thousands of years and is widely acknowledged as a topical agent for the relief of sunburn and skin irritations.

Digestive

The gel can be consumed (see contraindications above) when mixed with water or juice. The common preparation is to add two teaspoons of the clear aloe vera gel to a glass of water or fruit juice and drink before meals in order to reduce the severity of digestive problems. Alternatively, the aloe water or juice can be drunk after meals as a gentle remedy for heartburn. The juice is also very high in vitamin C and can help to lower blood sugar.

Laxative

The aloe vera juice has been shown to have the ability to act as a laxative to relieve constipation.

Skincare

The most widely recognized use for aloe vera is for skincare applications and is universally used for the care of sunburn. The gel is frequently used alone or incorporated into a salve as a face or hair moisturizer, which is especially recommended for dry, damaged, sensitive, or irritated skin or hair. It makes a particularly moisturizing overnight mask that can be used up to twice a week for extremely dry skin – apply the gel directly to the skin and leave overnight. Wash off in the morning with warm water. The aloe vera can also be used as a serum as part of your daily skin care regimen. Once the gel is extracted from the aloe leaves, add a little distilled water to reduce some of the stickiness from the gel and store it in a pump-top bottle to prevent contamination. Using aloe vera topically may help to reduce the appearance of dark spots and pigmentation. As will all skin preparations, it is important to test for allergic reactions when using aloe vera gel directly on the skin to ensure that there is no redness, rash, or irritation which could indicate an allergic reaction.

For the healing of sunburn, insect bites, or other skin irritations, a salve can be prepared ahead of time, or a leaf can be cut directly from the plant and the gel applied to the affected area. The gel soothes the skin, cooling it and speeding up the healing of sunburn as well as other types of burns. It will also soothe and speed healing of insect bites and other skin irritations.

Aloe vera salve can also be used as a personal lubricant and can be used in breastfeeding mothers to soothe sore nipples as an alternative to lanolin-based creams if a vegan option is preferred. If using the salve as a nipple cream, ensure that it is wiped off before nursing, as it does not taste great, and the baby may reject feeding.

Other Uses

Pure aloe gel, diluted aloe gel, or prepared salve can be applied to the hair before styling for smooth, shiny hair to reduce frizz and dandruff, and prevent hair loss. A mixture of aloe vera gel with water can also be used as a mouthwash to reduce dental plaque and to relieve bleeding or swollen gums.

Dosages:

> Aloe vera gel mixed with juice or water: up to three cups per day.
> Salve or pure aloe gel: Apply as needed.

Some folklore about aloe vera:

- Superstition states that if you grow aloe vera in the house, it will prevent household accidents, particularly burns.
- Another superstition suggests that aloe plants hung over doors of the house will bring luck and drive away evil.

-   It is said that Queen Cleopatra used aloe in her beauty routine.

Burdock (Arctium minus)

Properties: Antiinflammatory, Antioxidant, Decongestant, Diuretic, Expectorant.

Common Uses: Skin care issues, Digestive aid, Diuretic, Cough and Cold, Liver issues, high blood pressure.

Common Preparations: Tea, oil, tincture, pills, poultice, compress

Contraindications: Do not take internally if you are dehydrated or if you are taking any diuretic medication. Do not use externally if allergic to chrysanthemums or daisies. Do not take if pregnant, trying to become pregnant. Do not give to children under 12.

Burdock is considered safe to eat, but it is recommended not to gather from the wild, and to only gather or purchase from a reputable source as the burdock plant very closely resembles belladonna and nightshade plants which are very highly toxic, and these plants often grow close together.

Plant parts used: Root, seeds. Do not use the leaves internally.

Possible Side Effects

Burdock root may be associated with slow blood clotting and may increase the risk of bleeding in those with bleeding disorders.

Plant Identification

Burdock, also known as Gobo, grows around the world in wooded areas, and the plant is related to sunflowers and Daisies. The root is the part of the plant that is most often used, and it grows quite large, a two to three foot tuber, that has a woody, brown skin with white and fibrous flesh. The plant can grow up to four or five feet tall and has a stiff stem with a reddish color to it. Leaves are large and shaped like hearts with hairs on the undersides. Leaf edges can be wavy or can be toothed.

The plant is biannual, meaning that it takes two years to reach full maturity and flower. During the first year, the plant will remain as a rosette of leaves close to the ground. In the second year, a three to seven foot tall stalk will grow from the center of the leaf rosette and will grow purple flowers in July through October of the second year. The roots can be gathered from two-year-old plants in early spring, or from one-year-old plants in autumn. Leaves can be gathered throughout the year and used as needed. Flowers bloom in late summer, and fruits ripen in autumn. Collect the fruits when they are dry and stick to your clothing, then shake out the seeds. Lay seeds, roots, and leaves flat to dry.

The flowers are small and pink with a sweet fragrance, sitting on top of a seed ball. When the flowers dry, the seed balls turn brown and will stick to everything. In fact, the hooks on the burrs of burdock are reportedly the shape that inspired Velcro.

It is the root of burdock, which is made into tea and can be taken hot or cold. The root is harvested from the plant, sliced thinly, and then laid flat to dry completely. Once dried, the root is pulverized, and can then be used to make tea, salve, compress, and other preparations.

Historical Uses

Burdock root has a long history of use as a blood purifier, diaphoretic (increases sweating), and a diuretic. The root of the plant is linked with the ability to stimulate bile production and to regenerate cells of the liver.

Antiinflammatory

Burdock root has been shown to help in lowering blood pressure and opening blood vessels to improve blood flow. In cases of osteoarthritis, or even general aches and pains, the anti-inflammatory properties of the burdock root in the form of a salve or a compress can provide relief.

Antioxidant

Although they are not conclusive, there are some studies that suggest that the root of the burdock plant may contain some antioxidant properties which may help to prevent cancer cells from growing and mutating and even prevent some cancer cells from spreading. There are also some studies that suggest that the seeds of the burdock plant may also inhibit some cancers. More study is needed to confirm these claims, so it is best to consult with your healthcare provider before using burdock for this purpose.

Decongestant and Expectorant

Burdock root tea can be taken for relief of many respiratory issues. A tea made from burdock root can help to relieve the symptoms of coughs and colds as it is a decongestant as well as an expectorant that can clear the sinuses and lungs. Burdock does contain vitamin C as well, so it is likely is able to aid in boosting the immune system to fight off a cold.

Digestive Issues

When taken as a tea, burdock root can help to remove toxins from the blood, purifying it. It also acts as a digestive aid, strengthening and toning the stomach, and calming indigestion.

Diuretic

Diuretic agents promote urination and sweating and help to eliminate excess water weight. The tea made from decocting burdock root has been used to detoxify the liver for centuries, and can help reverse liver damage caused by alcohol consumption

Skincare

Burdock is commonly used for skincare issues, such as relieving bruises and inflammation. A poultice of the leaves can be used on the affected area as needed. For acne or eczema, a salve or compress can be applied to the affected area. The root also contains antioxidants, which fight free radicals and combat the signs of aging, such as wrinkles. For chronic skin diseases, use a tincture of the dried seeds to heal the skin from the inside out.

Other Uses

As well as its medicinal properties, Burdock root is also eaten as a vegetable in many cultures. In order to prepare the root for cooking, the outer layer must be peeled as it is quite bitter. The inner layer of the fresh root has a texture similar to a potato. Some popular preparations of burdock root include pickling the peeled root in vinegar, or slicing the roots into thin rounds, and then coating with olive oil and salt and roasting for about 25 minutes, flipping halfway through so both sides are browned.

Some use the tea or a tincture of burdock root to improve hair and scalp health, relieve dandruff, improve hair follicles to prevent hair loss, and improve hair thickness.

Dosages:

Tea: Up to three cups per day

Tincture 10-15 drops two to three times per day

Poultice: Apply twice per day, or as needed

Some folklore about Burdock:

- It is said that the inventor of Velcro, George de Mestral, got the idea for Velcro after removing dry burdock fruit from his dog's fur.
- Burdock has been used in several cultures to ward off negativity and for general protection.
- Some cultures consider burdock root to be an aphrodisiac.

Calendula (Calendula officinalis)

Properties: Antimicrobial, Antiinflammatory, Antiseptic

Common Uses: Wound healing, Soothing, Sunburn, Skincare, Skin irritations.

Common Preparations: Salve, Tea, Bath, Oil, Tincture, Pills, Compress

Contraindications: Avoid when pregnant since it can induce menstruation. Do not use if allergic to ragweed, daisies, marigold.

Plant parts used: Flowers

Possible Side Effects

Possible allergic reactions, including itching, rash, breathing problems, and dizziness. There is a possibility that it may cause a miscarriage if taken during pregnancy. May cause excessive drowsiness if taken during or after surgery. Consult a health care practitioner if you have an upcoming surgery.

Plant Identification

Also known as pot marigold, calendula is an annual plant that grows well in many environments and is known to attract butterflies. These flowers are similar, but not quite the same as the ornamental marigolds that are often grown alongside vegetable gardens (Tagetus genus). Calendula plants can grow as tall as two feet, and the flowers are a bright yellow to orange color. The flowers are usually between two to four inches in diameter, with the petals growing in two rows.

The petals of the calendula flower are known to reduce swelling and promote quicker healing when applied wounds and infections as a salve or a compress.   To harvest calendula, pick the flowers when they are at full bloom between early summer until the first frost of autumn. Deadheading the plant will cause the blooms to grow back and grow in fuller. The blooms should be harvested before they form seeds and laid on sheets in the sun to dry for about 2 weeks. The dried flowers can be stored in airtight containers if not prepared right away.

Historical Uses

Historically, calendula was used as a dye for fabrics and added to food such as butter and cheese to give it a yellow color. The blossoms have also been used in many rituals and ceremonies by the Romans and Greeks and Hindu cultures. Some of the earliest medicinal uses were topical treatments for skin conditions.

Antiinflammatory

As a pain reducer and antiinflammatory, it works well as a compress or salve for skin conditions such as diaper rash, eczema, dermatitis, and bacterial vaginosis. The salve used on the face can help to slow the development of wrinkles and reduce scarring.

Antibacterial/Antimicrobial

A tea of calendula petals can be used as a compress for eye infections. Using oil or salve on wounds or incisions can result in less healing time and faster healing, and it can be used to treat skin conditions, fight off infections, and prevent the growth of fungus, especially in the feet.

Menstruation

A tea of the dried petals is effective both for regulating an irregular or spotty flow and for inducing menstruation when the cycle has been interrupted. As such, should be avoided when pregnant.

Skin Issues

A bath or salve is safe for children and can be used on babies or children for skin irritations such as diaper rash, dry skin, eczema, insect bites, and any other type of skin irritation.

Muscle Relaxant

The salve can also be used to ease muscle spasms and soothe overworked muscles when massaged into the skin.

Cancer Treatments

There have been some studies to show that calendula tea and tincture can be used to treat the

side effects of cancer treatments, but there is inconclusive evidence, and more study is needed in this area.

Other Uses

The petals can also be used as a very effective dye. In past centuries, it has been used to dye cheeses and butter, and can also be used as a dye for fabric, giving natural fibers a light to medium yellow color. The flower petals can be eaten, and they have a mildly sweet and peppery flavor.

Dosages:

> Tincture: use 10 to 20 drops, up to three times per day.
> Salve, Bath, Compress: Use as needed.
> Tea: Add 2 teaspoons of dried flowers and steep 10 minutes. Can be taken once or twice daily.
> Pills: One or two pills daily as needed.

Some folklore about Calendula:

- Symbolizes the sun and used to decorate houses during celebrations.
- Also associated with death, since it is frequently located at graves because it will grow anywhere that there is a lot of sun.
- The petals have been traditionally used to dye fabrics and wool. Depending on the process used, calendula can produce anywhere from a light lemony yellow to olive, to a light brown. Herbal dyes work best on natural fibers, such as cotton or wool.

Chickweed (Stellaria media)

Properties: Antiinflammatory, Antipruritic, Astringent, Diuretic

Common Uses: Stomach and bowel problems, Joint pain, Menstrual pain, Respiratory illnesses.

Common Preparations: Poultice, Compress, Tea, Salve, Tincture

Contraindications: Can cause an allergic reaction, so it is best to avoid large amounts.

Plant parts used: Leaves, Stems, Flowers

Possible Side Effects

There are no real side effects reported from the use of chickweed, though it may cause allergic reactions in some people.

Plant Information

Chickweed is an annual plant that is generally considered a weed in North America. The mature plant has a hairy stem, oval leaves, and tiny daisy-like blossoms with ten petals. This herb has been used to treat wounds since the 16th century. It is important to note that there are several plants that look similar to chickweed, such as the mildly toxic yellow pimpernel, but one of the ways to identify chickweed is that it does not have milk sap like the others. Care should be taken when harvesting this herb in the wild. Products made from chickweed can be used internally or externally for several different health issues.

Unfortunately, chickweed does not keep well, and does not do well when refrigerated, so it is best to either use the fresh herb within a day of cutting it or dry it for future use.

Historical Uses

Chickweed has been used as a folk remedy for many different disorders, including blood issues, rheumatism, various types of inflammation, and skin problems including burns, and skin dryness due to eczema and psoriasis.

Antiinflammatory

One of the main uses for chickweed is to reduce swelling and treat inflammation, usually with a compress or poultice to the affected area. It has been found to be effective for the relief of pain from rheumatism, arthritis, and menstrual cramps. A poultice of the leaves can be applied for stomach and bowel problems, skin ulcers, muscle, and joint pain, or boils.

Antipruritic

A salve of chickweed flowers makes for a soothing massage and is useful for treating psoriasis as well as other dry skin disorders and can also be used as an anti-itch cream.

Astringent

A compress or a tincture has astringent properties, useful for drawing out splinters. As a skin treatment, they can be used to dry out acne, treat eczema, psoriasis, rashes, burns, and insect bites.

Diuretic

Chickweed tea may aid in weight loss, as a diuretic to help clean out the kidneys, and as digestive and intestinal support.

Culinary

The leaves of chickweed are high in vitamin C and can be cooked and eaten as a vegetable similar to spinach. The leaves are high in fiber and improve the absorption of nutrients, which leads to improved gut health. New growth in the spring is good in a salad. Chickweed can also be fed to livestock.

Dosages:

Tincture: Take 20 drops, one to three times daily.
Tea: One cup, once or twice daily.

Salve, Compress, Poultice: Apply as needed

Some folklore about Chickweed:

- English folklore regarding chickweed suggests that chickweed helps to maintain and strengthen relationships, and to encourage fidelity among lovers. Traditionally, a spring of chickweed was carried in order to catch a lover's eye and encourage them to be loyal.
- Is said to promote balance, since the plant itself seeks out soil with balanced conditions.
- The name of chickweed comes from the fact that it is often fed to baby chickens.
- Chickweed is connected with luck in Japan and is one of the seven herbs included in the symbolic porridge made for the festival of Nanakusa-no-sekku.

Dandelion (Taraxacum officinale)

Properties: Antidiabetic, Antiinflammatory, Antipruritic, Diuretic, Liver issues

Common Uses: Liver and gallbladder problems, diabetic issues, stomach and liver conditions

Common Preparations: Tea, Poultice, Tincture, Pills, Bath

Contraindications: Avoid if allergic to ragweed, chamomile, sunflowers, and daisies. May trigger a rash or other allergy symptoms. Do not use if allergic to iodine or latex. Avoid if pregnant, do not give to children. It is possible that excessive consumption may reduce fertility in both men and women.

There are several medications that may have adverse interactions with dandelion. The list includes antibiotics (Cipro and Penetrex), Antidepressants (Elavil), Antipsychotics (lithium and Haldol), Diuretics (Lasix), estrogen-based contraceptives. Check with health care professional.

Parts of plant used: Root, Leaves, Flower

Possible Side Effects

Dandelion root, leaves, and flowers are usually well tolerated by adults in moderation either as tea or as a food. Common side effects can include heartburn, diarrhea, upset stomach, irritated skin, muscle cramps, headache, dizziness, and changes in blood sugar.

Plant Identification

Dandelion is a common plant that is found around the world, and generally grows as a weed. The dandelion is universally recognizable with their jagged leaves, bright yellow flowers, and distinctive seed balls. They can grow in many climates from very warm to very cold climates, and generally bloom in May and June, but established plants can bloom again in September and October.

One drawback of foraging for dandelion is that it tends to absorb pesticides quite easily. Ensure that any dandelion that is harvested is growing away from roads, pesticides, pools, driveways, or any other sources of pollution. Once harvested, the roots must be dried completely to prevent mold, and then they can be stored for up to a year. Dried roots will be dark colored outside and have white insides.

Historical Uses

Dandelion has been used by Native American and Chinese healers for many years, mostly for liver and stomach conditions. The leaves have also been commonly used as a salad green or cooked, and is still used today in salads.

Antidiabetic Uses

Dandelion root contains a soluble fiber called inulin, which can help to support the growth of healthy bacteria in the gastrointestinal tract and help to eliminate the unhealthy bacteria. This slows the flow of sugar from the intestines to the bloodstream and prevents spikes in blood sugar or insulin levels and can help to regulate diabetes. There are also some studies that suggest that dandelion can stimulate pancreatic cells to produce insulin, which can help with controlling blood sugar and help avoid hyperglycemia. Dandelion tea can also be effective at calming prediabetic blood sugar spikes. It cannot take the place of prescribed diabetic medicine, and it is best to work with your healthcare provider if you wish to add dandelion to your diabetic regime.

If using dandelion for blood sugar issues, it is best to harvest the roots in the fall, when the inulin levels are at their highest.

Antiinflammatory

A poultice of the dried root can be helpful in treating various skin disorders, including acne, eczema, psoriasis, and boils due to its anti-inflammatory effect. There are many issues that the anti-inflammatory properties of dandelion may help with, including premenstrual bloating and water retention.

Antipruritic

Bathing in dandelion root can help to clear up skin disorders like acne, eczema, or any bacterial skin disorder and promote clear skin.

Diuretic

A tea made from dandelion roots tastes a little bit like coffee if the young roots are roasted until they are dark brown, then steeped and strained. This tea can help to eliminate excess water from the body and promote weight loss by breaking down fats and cholesterol.

Liver issues

It is generally thought that consuming dandelion flower tea will cleanse the liver, and studies show that dandelion root tincture can help to slow the progression of liver scarring. This allows the liver to heal and slowly regenerate.

Cancer

There are some studies that suggest that dandelion may help to prevent sun damage. The studies show that dandelion extracts are able to block UVB rays to some degree, which can protect the skin from sun damage and lower the risk of skin cancer. It is also possible that dandelion root may be able to be used as an anti-cancer agent for certain types of leukemia and melanoma. More study is needed.

Other Uses

Tea from the dried flowers can be helpful in cases of high cholesterol, heartburn, stomach disorders, promote strong bones, and may also protect against anemia.

Dosages:

Tincture: 10-15 drops taken two to three times per day.
Tea: One cup made from six to eight grams of fresh root or three to four grams of dried root, two to three times per day.
Salve, Compress, Poultice: Apply as needed

Some folklore about Dandelion:

- Once a dandelion has gone to seed, make a wish while you blow on the flower head, and the seeds will fly away and carry your wishes to make them come true.
- One superstition that has been around since medieval times is that if you hold a dandelion bloom under your chin, and your skin appears yellow, then you will be rich one day.
- Dandelions are traditionally woven into a wedding bouquet as a symbol of good luck for the newlyweds.

Echinacea (Echinacea purpurea)

Properties: Anti-
   inflammatory,
   Antioxidant,
   Immune-
   strengthening

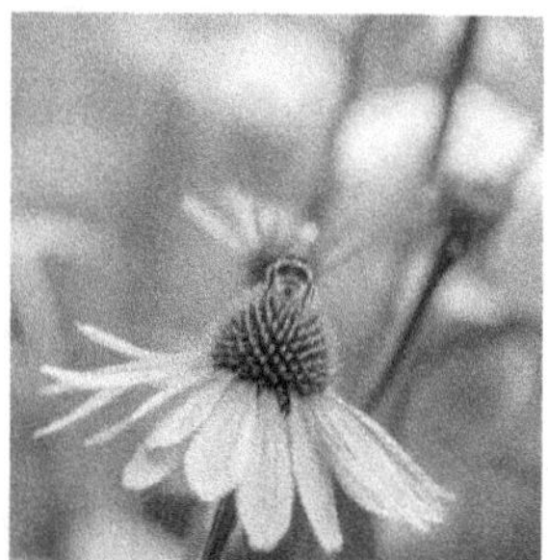

Common Uses: Alleviate
   pain, improve
   mental health,
   Relieve skin problems, Boost immunity

Common Preparations: Tea, Tincture

Contraindications: Do not use if pregnant or if
   suffering from asthma. Do not take if
   nursing. Do not use if taking
   immunosuppressant medications.

Part of plant used: Flower, Root, Leaves

Possible Side Effects

Echinacea is generally safe to take, though some of the side effects that have been rarely observed include nausea, vomiting, stomach pains, muscle or joint pain, headache, dizziness, confusion, and sleep problems. These side effects are rare, and echinacea is generally safe and well-tolerated by most people.

Plant Identification

Echinacea is a tall, purple, perennial plant with a cone-shaped flower, and is a member of the daisy family. It is also known by the name coneflower or purple coneflower. The stalk that the flower sits upon can grow up to four feet tall, and the flowers are between two to four inches in diameter. The plant grows well in many climates, though is native to the prairies and wooded areas of eastern and central North America. The plant can withstand drought, disease, insect infestations, is deer resistant, and is known to attract bees and butterflies to the garden.

The taste of echinacea is a mix between citrus and mint, and most people find it pleasing, though honey can be added to teas to make them more palatable if necessary.

Since the plant is perennial, the flowers can be harvested once they are at full bloom. Echinacea may or may not bloom during its first year, but it is important to wait until the plant has bloomed at least once before harvesting any part of it. Harvesting the root will effectively kill the plant, so it is best to wait until at least the third year so that you can get some use from the leaves and flowers first.

Historical Uses

The plant originated in North America and was used for many purposes by Native Americans for many years before it was adopted by Europeans in the 1800s.

Antiinflammatory

Because of anti-inflammatory properties, a compress or poultice has been used as a treatment for rheumatoid arthritis, ulcers, Chron's disease, and other conditions caused by inflammation, contributing to healing and relief.

Antioxidant

As an antioxidant, echinacea preparations can help with healthy cell growth. Echinacea can help to repair cells when taken internally by destroying the free radicals that can age and damage cells and has the potential to reduce or slow the growth of tumor cells according to some studies.

Respiratory Issues

Echinacea is usually prepared as a tea from the dried flowers and is used for easing respiratory issues such as bronchitis. A bath from echinacea may also be helpful for respiratory issues.

Immune-Strengthening

Echinacea is proven to boost immunity and can be effective at shortening the duration of flu symptoms and can even reduce the odds of getting a cold by up to 58%. It has been shown to strengthen the immune system by increasing the production of white blood cells to help fight viruses and bacteria and reduce the severity and duration of colds and possibly flus as well.

Anxiety

Echinacea tea is sometimes recommended for those who suffer from ADHD to relieve anxiety, depression, and social phobia. Echinacea can help to regulate the communication between the body and the brain in order to help to instill a feeling of calm and quiet, and to reduce anxiety.

Blood Sugar Issues

Echinacea can also be used to control blood sugar. It can help to keep blood sugar from spiking in those with diabetes or prediabetes. It can keep blood sugar from plummeting if hypoglycemic, though it is not a replacement for insulin or other diabetes treatments. The components in echinacea are alcohol-soluble, so it may be more potent when taken as a tincture rather than a tea.

Other Uses

Echinacea can also be used as a treatment against many types of infections, including urinary tract infections, herpes, vaginal yeast infections, nose and throat infections, and even warts.

Dosages:

> Tea from roots or flowers: two to three cups of tea to keep the immune system healthy, and up to five cups per day when sick. One to two cups of tea per day to help with blood sugar, blood pressure, or anxiety.
> Bath or salve: As needed

Some folklore about Echinacea:

- In addition to attracting bees and butterflies, echinacea is also said to attract flower fairies to the garden.
- Native Americans used echinacea as an offering to spirits and to strengthen rituals.

Elder (Sambucus nigra)

Properties: Anti-inflammatory, Antioxidant, Diuretic, Laxative

Common Uses of Berries: Lower blood sugar, stop bleeding, colds and flu, treat infections, sciatica, headache, dental pain, heart and nerve pain, laxative

Common Uses of Flowers: Pain relief, swelling, inflammation, diuretic, induce sweating

Bark: diuretic, laxative, induce vomiting

Common Preparations: Tea, Syrup, Compress, Poultice, Culinary, Bath, Tincture

Contraindications: Raw berries, bark, and leaves are toxic and can cause stomach problems. Not recommended for children, or for pregnant women. Stop using elderflower products 2 weeks before any surgery to avoid possible complications.

Plant parts used: Flowers, Berries, Bark.

Possible Side Effects

Nausea and vomiting are possible if the raw berries are eaten. When using any elder products, possible side effects can include weakness, dizziness, or numbness.

Plant Identification

The elder shrub or tree can grow up to 30 feet tall, so it is much larger than many commonly used herbs. It tends to grow the best in rich, damp soil on riverbanks and other wet areas. The flowers bloom in clusters with dozens of small white flowers coming from a central stalk, and bloom in May or June. The flowers can be harvested by cutting just below where the flower stalks converge, but make sure not to harvest all of the flowers; otherwise, no berries will grow on the tree. The tree's berries are about five to seven millimeters in diameter and purple to black in color. The berries ripen in September and must be harvested quickly because they are a favorite of songbirds and can disappear overnight when ripe. It is said that elderberry and elderflower are the oldest herbs cultivated and used by humans.

The berries need to be cooked before they can be eaten, but the flowers can be consumed raw or cooked. There are many species of elder, but American or European elderberry are the safest to use, and other species may have more toxic effects. Bark, unripe berries, and seeds can cause stomach problems and should not be ingested raw in large amounts, if at all. Cooking neutralizes the toxins in the berries.

Both berry tincture and tea from the flowers can reduce the severity and length of a cold or flu.

They can shrink swollen sinuses, inhibit the growth of bacteria, and improve the symptoms of

Sinusitis, bronchitis, and coughs. Additionally, a lozenge made from the berries or flowers has been shown to reduce the flu symptoms of fever, headache, muscle ache, and nasal congestion.

Historical Uses

Native American healers used berries to treat infection, ancient Egyptians used elder preparations for burns and to improve complexion.

Anti-inflammatory

An elderflower compress or bath can help to stop the flow of blood to a wound, reduce bruising, and to reduce swelling. A salve can be massaged into the joints, or a warm compress can be applied to ease the pain of arthritis.

Antioxidant

The berries, leaves, and flowers of the elder all have well documented antioxidant properties, and the berries may contain some cancer-inhibiting properties and support the immune system by increasing white blood cells.

Blood Sugar

Elder has been used for many years to help to lower blood sugar, but care must be taken for those with diabetes since it can adversely interact with diabetes medication, and there is a danger that it may lower blood sugar too far. Elder preparations have shown to be able to increase insulin secretion and improve blood sugar levels, but it is best to work with your healthcare provider if you are being treated for diabetes.

Culinary

In cooking, elderflower is a popular flavoring in drinks and desserts. Elderflower syrup can be found in many cocktails, and sodas. The berries are commonly harvested to make juice, jams, pies, or wine. Both the berries and the flowers contain high concentrations of vitamins A, B, C, and E.

Diuretic

A tea or syrup made from the flowers can help to ease constipation and to increase urine production.

Skincare

In skincare, a bath of elderflower is used to tighten skin and improve the complexion, including fading freckles, age spots, and blemishes. A compress or a salve of elderflower may be used as a facial mask treatment one or two times per week in order to refresh the complexion. It is a mild astringent and is good for mature skin.

Other Uses

The extract of elderflowers is also used frequently in perfumes, and its scent has been described as sweet, honey, herbal, spicy.

Dosages:

> Syrup: One tablespoon of berry or flower syrup four times per day.
> Tea: Up to three cups per day.
> Compress, poultice, bath, salve: As needed.

Some folklore about Elder:

- It is said that if you dream of elderberries, then you will become sick soon.
- An elder tree growing near a home will protect all who live in the home.
- In German folklore, it is believed that anyone who injures an elder tree will suffer from its vengeance.
- In the middle ages, the leaves were used to ward off witches, and the berries were placed on the windowsills to repel vampires.

- It is believed that if you stand under an elder tree at midnight on midsummer, you will see the fairies.

Marshmallow (Althaea officinalis)

Properties: Analgesic,   Anti-inflammatory, Antioxidant, Diuretic

Common Uses: Digestive, Respiratory, Skin conditions, Cough, and cold.

Common Preparations: Syrup, Pill, Tincture, Tea, Salve, Oil

Contraindications: Avoid   if   pregnant, breastfeeding, or diabetic. Do not use if surgery is scheduled in the next 2 weeks.

Parts of plant used: Root, Leaf, Flower

Possible side effects

Possible side effects include upset stomach and dizziness. Root preparations should only be taken for four weeks at a time, then a one week break before resuming use. Skin applications have the potential for skin irritation. Do a patch test before applying to a large area.

Plant Identification

Marshmallow is an annual plant that typically grows to about three to four feet high. The leaves are small, about two to three inches long, and vaguely resemble the shape of a maple leaf with five points. The flowers resemble a wild rose and are a light pink color. The flowers bloom in late summer, so they are harvested then. The leaves and roots of the plant are also used and can be harvested all year round. The plant prefers slightly sandy soil and grows well on riverbanks and in salt marshes. The marshmallow is native to Europe but has been found in North and South America since colonization.

The marshmallow has a unique gooey texture, and this makes it especially well-suited for preparations that are meant to coat the throat or stomach. The root of the marshmallow plant contains the sap that was used to make sweet marshmallow candy as a food product originally, though commercially prepared marshmallows are no longer made from the marshmallow plant.

Historical Uses

The marshmallow plant, especially the root, has been used for thousands of years in Egypt and Asia for digestive, respiratory, and skin conditions. The name "Althaea" comes from the Greek word for 'to heal.'

Analgesic and Antiinflammatory

Marshmallow has antiinflammatory properties and wound healing properties, and a salve applied can provide some pain relief and can dramatically reduce swelling. Since it is also soothing to the skin, it will also help any wounds to heal more quickly and lessen the appearance of any scars.

Antioxidant

There are some suggestions that a tincture of marshmallow leaves and flowers can help to protect the body from damage of free radicals, which may help to prevent certain cancers. In addition, preparations of the root may stimulate cells and support tissue regeneration.

Digestive Issues

A tea made from marshmallow root contains an enzyme that helps to loosen mucous and inhibit bacterial growth. It can ease an upset stomach, constipation, or diarrhea, as well as soothing irritation and inflammation of the digestive tract.

Diuretic

Drinking a few cups of marshmallow root tea throughout the day can help to cleanse the kidneys and bladder by flushing out excess liquid and can clear up urinary infections.

Respiratory Issues

Syrup from marshmallow root can help to clear mucus membranes, or syrup from the flowers makes a good expectorant for coughs. Lozenges can help to soothe a dry cough and irritated throat.

Skincare

Marshmallow root applied as a tincture or as a compress topically can help to calm many skin problems, such as acne, as well as inflamed skin from cuts and scrapes. A compress or a poultice from the leaves can also be applied to bruises in order to heal them faster. A salve or a bath of marshmallow root helps to maintain the skin's natural moisture level and promote overall skin health.

Blend a few large marshmallow leaves with some mineral water in the blender and apply to the face to draw out impurities, especially of acne. Can be used a few times per week, and will leave the skin smooth and bright.

Other uses

Marshmallow leaves can be eaten raw in a salad or can be cooked as well. For vegans looking for an egg substitute, the gooey liquid produced by boiling the marshmallow plant creates the right consistency for a substitution, though it is bright green and will turn your baking green.

Dosage

>Tea: Two to three cups per day.
>Salve, Compress, Poultice: Apply as needed.
>Tincture: 20-40 drops, three times per day
>Syrup: Two tablespoons of cough syrup per day.

Some folklore about Marshmallow:

- Celtic people would place the flat seed disks of the marshmallow over the eyes of the dead to prevent evil spirits from sneaking into the body for a free ride to heaven.
- A piece of marshmallow root worn in the shoe will lead the wearer to buried treasure.

Mullein (Verbascum Thapsus)

Properties: Antibacterial, Antiinflammatory, Antiviral

Common Uses: Respiratory, antiinflammatory, skincare, ear pain

Common Preparations: Tea, Syrup, Tincture, Poultice, Compress, Salve, Oil

Contraindications: Avoid if pregnant or breastfeeding.

Part of plant used: Leaves, flower

Possible Side Effects

There are no reports of major side effects, although the mullein plant has tiny hairs on the leaves and stalk, which can cause skin irritation when raw. When making tea, the liquid must be strained thoroughly after steeping and before drinking so the hairs do not irritate the throat.

Plant Identification

Mullein grows well in environments with little rainfall and grows well in disturbed landscapes. Mullein is biennial, meaning that it has a 2-year growing cycle. In its first year, it forms a small rosette of hairy or velvety leaves that can be up to 12 inches long. In the second year of growth, a flower stalk will grow in the center of the leaves and can be up to 6 feet tall. The entire stalk is covered with hairs, which can be very irritating to the skin. The leaves are known as 'bunny ears' because of their soft, velvet-like appearance.

The flowers of the mullein are pale yellow with five petals, and each can measure approximately ¼ inch to 1 inch across. The flowers are arranged in a cluster at the top of the stalk in a club-like shape, and blooms from June to September. The flowers bloom depending on the weather conditions, so there may be some years where the mullein does not bloom at all. It is very rare for all of the flowers to bloom at once. Usually, a few flowers will bloom on the spike, then they will die and produce seeds and another few flowers will bloom. If harvesting flowers from the mullein, check every few days to harvest what is there.

Historical Uses

In the late 1800s, tea was a popular treatment for tuberculosis. There is also some evidence that the leaves may have been smoked in an effort to calm respiratory ailments. There are historical records which show that the leaves were used by Native Americans and American colonists in their shoes to keep out the cold, and even some records that show that the leaves were used as toilet paper. It is not clear how this is handled with the potentially irritating nature of the hairs, so is not recommended.

Antibacterial and Antiviral

Mullein has been shown to have antibacterial properties and to inhibit the growth of several strains of bacteria that can cause infection. It also has some antiviral properties and can reduce the severity and treat the symptoms of respiratory issues, including tuberculosis, tonsillitis, bronchitis, and even pneumonia. There is also possible evidence that it may be able to fight influenza A and herpes as well, though this information is not well documented and more study is required.

Respiratory

For hundreds of years, a tea of the mullein flowers and leaves has been used to treat respiratory conditions such as cough, congestion, cold, and asthma. It is particularly good at relieving asthma because it can reduce swelling in the airway, and therefore can reduce the symptoms of coughing, wheezing, and shortness of breath. It does not, however, replace asthma medications, so care must be taken to consult your healthcare practitioner if you are using any medications for asthma before adding mullein to your healthcare regime.

Anti-inflammatory

The anti-inflammatory properties of mullein flowers and leaves that are helpful for the respiratory tract can also be used for other inflammation issues in the body. Mullein oil or compress can be used to calm any areas of inflammation or joint pain. The flowers and leaves of mullein in a tea, compress, poultice, or salve can be used for headache or migraine or for pain anywhere in the body. The tea also works well for relieving constipation and gout.

Ear Pain

For ear pain and ear infections, a compress of mullein flowers and leaves may be applied to the ear to relieve ear pain, especially in children. Make sure that the compress is warm, replace it when it cools off. Make sure that the cloth is rung out so that there is no liquid entering the ear canal.

Other Uses

After the growing season was over, the stalk was often cut, dried, and then the tip dipped in wax. The resulting stalk can be used as a torch and once dipped in wax burns for quite a long time. The dried leaves and stem can also be used for a very good tinder.

The flowers can be boiled to produce a bright yellow dye for dying cloth. Adding a basic agent (raising the pH) will produce a brown dye, and adding an acid (lowering the pH) will produce a green dye.

Dosages:

> Tea: One to two cups daily made from flowers or leaves.
> Compress, poultice, or salve: As needed
> Oil (external only): As needed

Some folklore about Mullein:

- In medieval England, the mullein was used to determine whether a lover was faithful. The plant was bent towards the lover's house. If it resumed a vertical position, then all was well, but if it died, then the lover was untrue.
- Mullein was considered to be a sure safeguard against evil spirits and magic.

Nettle (Urtica dioica)

Properties: Anti-inflammatory, Antioxidant, Galactagogue

Common Uses: Culinary, Allergy relief, Blood pressure, Kidney, and bladder issues.

Common Preparations: Tea, Salve, Tincture, Culinary

Contraindications: Do not take nettles if also taking blood thinners, blood pressure medication, diuretics, diabetes medication, or lithium. Do not take when pregnant as there is a danger of miscarriage.

Parts of plant used: Leaves and flowers.

Possible Side Effects

Leaves can cause a temporary burning sensation on contact. If fresh nettle does come in contact with the skin, it can cause a raised bumpy rash, which is quite itchy. In rare cases, it can cause tightness in the chest or throat, breathing difficulty, wheezing, swelling in the mouth, tongue, or lips, stomach cramps, vomiting, or diarrhea. In the case of a rash, make sure not to touch the affected area for at least 10 minutes. Any rubbing or touching of the area can push the chemicals deeper into the skin and make them more difficult to remove and make the rash more difficult to relieve. After the irritation has rested for 10 minutes, use soap and water to gently wash away the nettle's chemicals from the surface of the skin. Often the pain will be relieved when the skin is washed.

If there are still some of the nettle hairs stuck in the skin. The best way to get rid of them is to place some adhesive tape over the affected area, and then pull it loose, similar to waxing. If the above method does not fully relieve the effects of the sting, try a compress of cool water or aloe vera juice, salve, or pure aloe gel.

If the rash does not disappear after 24 hours, then it is likely a more severe allergic reaction, and you should consult a healthcare professional.

Plant Identification

Nettle is a shrub that is found worldwide. The plant is perennial and can grow to between three to seven feet tall in the summer, dying down to nothing in the winter. The leaves are strongly serrated and are attached on opposite sides of a hairy stem. The stems and leaves have hairs, some of which can inject chemicals into the skin and cause a stinging sensation. Wear long pants, long sleeves, and gloves when harvesting nettle.

The flowers are small and can be either greyish yellow or greyish green and hairy. The flowers bloom between May to September.

Historical Uses

Nettle has been used for arthritis and lower back pain since ancient Egyptian times. Roman troops would rub the herb on their skin to give them the illusion of warmth in cold climates.

Anti-inflammatory

Nettle has great anti-inflammatory properties, and tea, pills, salve, or compress are all useful ways to reduce inflammation and pain from arthritis. Tea or tincture may help to treat the symptoms of an enlarged prostate or other urinary problems.

Antioxidant

There is evidence that shows that a nettle tincture can defend against free radicals, which are linked to aging, cancer, and other diseases.

Culinary

Nettles have long been eaten as a nutritious vegetable. Once they have been processed, dried, or cooked, nettle can be safely consumed and is very nutritious, containing high levels of vitamins A, C, K, calcium, iron, and magnesium.

Allergies

Nettle tea can help to treat hayfever by blocking histamine receptors and reducing inflammation in the lining of the nose, relieving seasonal allergies

Blood Pressure

Preparations of nettle have proven helpful in lowering blood pressure and the risk of heart disease and stroke. It acts as a calcium channel blocker, which relaxes the heart muscles by reducing the force of the contractions and stimulating nitric oxide production, which can relax the muscles of the blood vessels and help them widen.

Kidney and Bladder Problems

As a diuretic, nettle tea may help to remove excess salt and water from the body, helping to relieve the symptoms of kidney and bladder stones, and also of urinary tract infections.

Other Uses

Native Americans used the fiber from the nettle to make fishing nets and cord. This fiber can still be used today to create a fabric similar to linen. The leaves can produce a green dye that was used in wartime Europe to make camouflage.

Dosages:

> Tea: Two to three cups per day.
> Tincture: One to two milliliters taken up to three times per day.
> Salve, compress: As needed.

Some folklore about Nettle:

- Old English folklore says that girls should gather nettles early on the morning of May first, boil them in water, and then use the nettle water to rinse their hair so that it will grow long and strong.
- "Nettling" or "urtication" is a tradition where each person holds a bundle of nettles and gently whips everyone in the home in order to awaken their agility and protect them against illness.

Oats (Avena sativa)

Properties: Cardiovascular, Nervine, Skin disorders

Common Uses: Anxiety, bladder weakness, constipation, diverticulosis, gout, inflammatory bowel disease, IBS, joint and tendon disorders, kidney conditions, nerve disorders, gallstones, skin disorders, stress, dermatitis, pruritis, acne, eczema.

Common Preparations: Bath, Salve, Tea, Tincture, Poultice, Culinary

Contraindications: Do not take if diagnosed with celiac disease or disorder of digestive tract, intestinal obstruction, digestive disorders that slow down the digestive process. Do not give topically to children with atopic dermatitis as it may trigger an allergic reaction.

Parts of plants used: Immature seeds, mature seeds, stem, leaves

Possible Side Effects

Oats are generally considered to be safe to give to anyone, including babies, the elderly, and pregnant women.   The only major contraindication is for those with celiac disease or gluten intolerance, for which the side effects can include gas or bloating when taken internally. It is felt that the oats can still be used topically in those with gluten intolerance, but it would be best to perform a skin test prior to using any preparation containing oat just to be sure that there will not be an allergic reaction.

Plant Identification

Oat is a cereal grain that is grown all over the world and used as a staple food crop. The main part of the plant that is used commercially is the seed, and this is the bag of oats that you will see at the grocery store.

Oats grow from a stalk that is about two to three feet tall when mature. Oats grow quite quickly and will usually be ripe about 12 weeks after planting. They are ready for harvest once the seed heads turn from green to a light brown or cream color. The immature seed, called milky oats because they ooze a milky white liquid, can be harvested in the early part of the growth cycle. These immature seeds contain the highest amounts of magnesium and potassium.

The dried mature seeds are the seeds that are most commonly used as food.

The stems and leaves of the oat plant can also be harvested and dried. This is called oat straw, and can be made into a tea

Historical Uses

Milky oats were often made into a gruel have been used historically for those suffering from malnutrition, diarrhea, or dysentery. Oatmeal has long been a staple of the diets of those who needed a boost to their nutrition, or who had limited access to proper nutrition. Most skin disorders have been treated by an oat preparation at some point due to its cooling and soothing properties.

Cardiovascular

Eating oats has been shown to help to lower the amount of fats in the blood and to reduce the risk of, or even prevent heart disease, and can lower blood pressure.

Skin Disorders

Oats soothe itch, combat skin dryness and oiliness, calm eczema, and contact dermatitis. They can also help to absorb and remove oil and bacteria from the skin, exfoliate dead skin cells.

As a compress, poultice, or a bath, oats work wonders in soothing eczema and other skin conditions, especially if the skin is dry or itchy. A poultice applied as a face mask for acne can help to calm the swelling and redness and speed the healing of acne. A warm oat bath can calm the itching of poison ivy, chickenpox, or sunburn.

Addiction Issues

Taking a tincture of oats can help to reduce the craving for nicotine, and also help with withdrawal from nicotine and narcotics.

Gastrointestinal Disorders

All preparations of oats can increase the gut flora and help to relieve abdominal pain, including eating them as oatmeal. There are some studies which show that there are possibilities for oats to help to prevent gallstones, and some cancers, including colon and stomach, but not a lot of research has been done to support these claims.

Nervous Disorders

Oats have proven to be both soothing and calming to help rebuild the nervous system when eaten, or when taken as a tea, tincture, or as a bath. A tincture can be taken to improve attention, concentration, increase energy, and ability to maintain focus, mood, and calm. It is good for relieving anxiety and stress. overcoming exhaustion, and helping restore normal nerve function,

Culinary

Oats contain high amounts of fiber and are very nourishing for those who are malnourished or undernourished. Eating oats regularly can help to prevent joint pain and rheumatism, help combat fatigue, and can also be helpful in the treatment of diarrhea and constipation. Oats are commonly eaten before a workout for more endurance and prolonged energy.

Other Uses

A bowl of oats in the fridge or freezer will help to absorb bad odors from food. Oats are also safe to use as a compress or bath for dogs with itchy, dry skin.

Dosages:

Tincture: 10-20 drops, once or twice per day.
Poultice, compress, bath: As needed
Tea: one to two cups per day as needed.

Some folklore about Oats:

- When oats fail, it is a sure sign that other grains will have poor harvests as well.
- Oats are associated with prosperity.

Peppermint (Mentha piperita)

Properties: Antibacterial, Carminative, Digestive, Nervine

Common Uses: Headache, stomach upset, and digestive issues, anxiety.

Common Preparations: Tea, Compress, Pills, Culinary

Contraindications: Do not get in eyes, may irritate mucous membranes.

Plant parts used: Leaves

Possible Side Effects

Peppermint is generally safe for all people, but in very rare cases, there can be allergic reactions, headache, or rash observed.

Plant Identification

The peppermint plant grows in almost every climate and is sometimes considered an invasive species because it tends to spread widely when not tightly controlled. Herb gardeners will often grow it in pots to prevent it from taking over the whole garden. The plant itself is a perennial plant that can be between 20-30 inches tall when mature. Leaves are dark green, about three to four inches long and about two inches wide. The leaves end in a sharp point and have toothed margins. The plants grow well in most habitats, and as mentioned above, grow quickly and spread out over a wide area if allowed.

The leaves should be harvested in spring or early summer before the flowers grow, or they will taste bitter. The flowers are small and purple and grow in mid to late summer.

Historical Uses

Peppermint has been used for many centuries by various cultures for its medicinal value. It has been written about in ancient Greek myths, by the Roman naturalist Pliny the Elder, and in Icelandic medical documents from the 13th century. It has been used in Europe since the 18th century. It has been reported that peppermint was used in Europe to whiten teeth as far back as the 14th century, as well as being used to mask the smell of tobacco.

Antibacterial

Drinking the tea from peppermint leaves or using the oil on the skin can help to fight bacterial infections, killing bacteria, and helping to prevent the growth of food-borne bacteria. Peppermint has been shown to kill several types of bacteria that can cause illness in humans, including bacteria that lead to pneumonia, and it also kills mouth bacteria that can lead to gingivitis, and so is added to many mouthwash preparations.

Carminative/ Digestive

A tea from peppermint leaves can be taken before eating in order to avoid gas pains, or it can be taken after a meal to help with indigestion. The calming and soothing actions of the peppermint herb aids in digestion, relieves indigestion, eases nausea, and can help with calming other gastrointestinal issues. The tea soothes the stomach wall and can help to ease nausea and prevent vomiting felt during pregnancy and caused by motion sickness. The tea is commonly used to relieve digestive issues such as gas, bloating, indigestion, and can improve the symptoms of irritable bowel syndrome.

Nervine

Drinking peppermint tea has been shown to relieve anxiety and help patients to maintain focus. Taking pills may help to increase energy and reduce the incidence of daytime sleepiness in the long term.

Headache

One of the most widely recognized uses for peppermint is as a treatment for headaches. For a headache or a migraine, placing a compress of peppermint or peppermint oil over the headache, or on the temples and forehead can provide a cooling sensation and increase blood flow, which in turn can help to ease the pain.

Allergies and Sinus Issues

The antibacterial, antiviral, and anti-inflammatory properties of peppermint tea can help to relieve clogged sinuses, shrinking them and therefore improving air flow. It can also help to reduce the symptoms of seasonal allergies, such as runny nose, itchy eyes, and even to alleviate some of the symptoms of asthma.

Muscle Relaxant

As a tea or compress or pill, peppermint can be very helpful in relieving menstrual cramps or applied topically as a salve can relieve any sore muscles or muscle fatigue. The muscle relaxant properties have also been reported to help with relaxation before bed. However, it is also reported to increase energy, so caution must be used if intending to use peppermint for this purpose.

Other Usages

Inhaling the steam from a tea, oil, or even the fresh leaves can help to Improve concentration and may improve memory and alertness. Peppermint is widely acknowledged as a breath freshener and has antibacterial properties that can kill various bacteria that can cause dental plaque. Removal of this dental plaque can improve breath. Greeks and Romans used peppermint to flavor sauces and wines, and it was commonly used to scent bath water and bedding.

Dosages:

Bath, Salve, Compress, Poultice: As needed
Tea: one to three cups per day
Tincture: up to 20 drops taken three times per day for up to 8 weeks.

Some folklore about Peppermint:

- Mint was used in Assyrian rituals to their fire god.
- Greeks and Romans wore crowns of mint at feasts.
- Traditionally an herb of hospitality.

Plantain (Plantago major)

Properties: Analgesic, Antibacterial, Antiinflammatory, Antiseptic, Astringent.

Common Uses: Relieve pain, Staunch bleeding, fight infection, soothe inflammation, relieve itching.

Common Preparations: Tea, Bath, Salve, Culinary, Compress, Poultice.

Contraindications: Don't use internally if blood disorder or prone to blood clots. Do not take if pregnant or breastfeeding.

Parts of Plant Used: leaves, seeds

Possible Side Effects

Plantain is considered to be a safe herb to take for most adults. Rare possible side effects include low blood pressure and diarrhea. In some cases, applying plantain to the skin may cause an allergic reaction such as itching or rash.

Plant Identification

Plantain is a perennial plant with oval-shaped leaves that are approximately six to eight inches long and three inches wide. The leaves grow in a rosette close to the ground, and can grow in many climates, but are most commonly found along roadsides, fields, or other areas that have been disturbed by humans. The flowers are small and green to brown and grow in a dense spike that can be up to six inches long on the top of a six-inch stem, making the full height of the plant 12 inches.

Since the plant survives well in disturbed and damaged areas, it have proven to be a useful plant to help soil rehabilitation. The roots help to break up hard soils and can help to make the soils more habitable for other plants in the future. Somewhat different from other plants, the leaves of the plantain are the most medically potent when the flowers are in bloom.

Historical Uses

There is a legend that the plantain was discovered by Alexander the great and brought to Europe in 327 BCE. In North America, plantain was called Whiteman's Footprint by the Native Americans since they perceived that it seemed to spring up wherever the white men went. Plantain was also considered one of the nine sacred herbs of the Saxons, and was an early Christian symbol of the path followed by the devout.

Analgesic

The leaves can be used fresh as an analgesic. Bruise or cut the leaves and then apply them directly to a wound or cut for pain relief. A salve of the leaves, a compress, or an herbal oil can also be applied for pain relief purposes.

Antibacterial

The antibacterial properties of plantain are well documented. A salve, compress, or oil used on cuts and bruises can speed the recovery of wounds and act as an antibacterial agent to prevent the wound from spreading.

Antiinflammatory

Used as a tea of the leaves, plantain can help to soothe internal membranes, including relief from diarrhea. A tea of the root of the plantain can help to reduce swelling in respiratory tissues and aid in the healing of respiratory infections. Taking a bath of plantain is uplifting, cooling, and refreshing, but can also help to relieve nasal and chest congestion through reducing swelling of the nasal passages.

A plantain compress, poultice, or bath can soothe inflammation resulting from bites, stings, rashes, eczema, psoriasis, burns, cuts, varicose veins. A tea or tincture can provide hemorrhoid relief over time, relieve IBS, constipation, diarrhea, indigestion, and ulcers. Fresh leaves can be bruised so that some of the juices come out, and then applied topically to treat insect bites, stings, eczema, small wounds, cuts, inflamed skin, or dermatitis.

Antiseptic

A poultice of plantain leaves works to facilitate healing and prevent infection to wounds, stings, and sores. It has been shown to promote cellular growth and tissue regeneration. Plantain root also works well for respiratory infections.

Astringent

As an astringent, plantain can speed the recovery of wounds. A compress or a salve from the leaves helps to soothe mosquito bites and other types of bites and stings by helping to draw the poison or venom out from the skin. It is also quite helpful to draw splinters out from the skin.

A tea of plantain leaves is used to treat diarrhea and soothe internal membranes. A compress applied to a sunburn or a rash from poison ivy, poison oak, or sumac will draw out the poison and relieve the itch. It has also been used to numb the skin, which also helps with sunburn, dermatitis, or injury. It has been used effectively to numb the skin as a compress applied before piercing, tattooing, or hair removal procedures to help reduce the swelling or pain from the procedure.

Digestive

Plantain tea can be used to help regulate cholesterol and diabetes, and to calm indigestion and heartburn.

Culinary

Plantain has been eaten as a leaf vegetable for many years, and is very high in vitamins C. K. A, as well as calcium and beta-carotene. The fresh, young spring leaves taste the best as the older the leaves get, they get stringy and can have a stronger flavor. The older leaves are great for making tea or other preparations but are less palatable for culinary purposes.

Heart Health

Some sources indicate that the seeds of the plantain plant may lower cholesterol when ingested, and a tea from the seeds is useful for many heart ailments.

Other Uses for Plantain

The flower spikes can be harvested and dried then given to caged birds. Swishing plantain tea or a diluted tincture can help to heal mouth ulcers and prevent infections in the mouth.

Dosages:

     Tincture: up to 10 drops, three times per day
     Tea: one to three cups per day
     Salve, Compress, Poultice: As needed

Some folklore about Plantain:

- One of the Saxon's 'Nine Sacred Herbs.'
- Often called 'White Man's Footprint' by Native Americans because it seemed to sprout wherever Europeans spent time in North America.

Red Clover (Trifolium pretense)

Properties: Antiinflammatory, Antioxidant

Common Uses: Respiratory issues, skin disorders, inflammatory conditions, women's health problems.

Common Preparations: Tea, Tincture, Compress, Poultice

Contraindications: Do not use if pregnant or breastfeeding. Do not use if you have a hormone-sensitive cancer. Do not use if taking methotrexate.

Plant Parts Used: Flowers, leaves can be used as well.

Possible Side Effects

Red clover is safe for short term use, but not recommended for long-term or regular use because of the possible link to risk of cancer in the uterus lining. Too much can be toxic

It should not be used for longer than three to six months without consulting a healthcare provider. Red clover has blood-thinning ability and can increase the effect of antiplatelet and anticoagulant drugs. Do not take if on blood thinners.

Plant Identification

Red clover belongs to the legume family along with peas and beans. It is a perennial herbaceous plant with small leaflets that grow most often in groupings of three and are green with a white chevron mark on them. The plant grows to about 16 inches tall, and the flower blooms from early June and July. The flowers grow in a distinctive pink/purple ball that is about one inch in diameter. The flower ball is actually a cluster of up to 100 florets growing from the same stem.

It is usually the flowers that are used, but flowers and leaves can both be harvested for medicinal preparations. In the garden, red clover is able to fix atmospheric nitrogen in the soil and make it biologically available for other plants, which makes it a good plant neighbor.

Historical Uses

In Europe, red clover has been used as a medicinal herb for hundreds of years to treat liver and digestive ailments. Native American cultures have used it as a salve for burns, for eye issues, and as a vegetable.

Antiinflammatory

Red clover has been used for Inflammatory conditions for many years. It has properties which can help to alleviate the symptoms of arthritis and rheumatism when taken as tea and can also be used as a salve and rubbed into the skin for relief of inflammation, rash, and irritation.

Antioxidant

Antioxidants in the leaves and petals of red clover can be used as a tea to help neutralize free radicals, and so can prevent degenerative diseases and cell mutation. Drinking the tea may reduce the risk of prostate cancer because of the estrogen-like effects, but conversely may increase the risk of estrogen cancers such as breast cancer and endometrial cancer. Studies have shown encouraging evidence of red clover as a supplemental treatment for cancers but should not be used for breast cancer since it has estrogen-like properties. It is best to consult with a healthcare practitioner.

Respiratory Issues

For respiratory issues such as asthma, whooping cough, and bronchitis, a tea, bath, or compress to the chest of red clover is recommended. Red clover tea is also often used for children with a persistent cough and is well tolerated by children because of the honey-like flavor. The clover can also be made into a syrup for administering to patient with a cough.

Skin Disorders

A bath of red clover or a compress to the affected area can be helpful in skin disorders such as eczema and psoriasis, reducing inflammation and calming itch.

Heart and Blood Issues

One of the more widespread uses of red clover is for heart and blood issues. Red clover tea can reduce the tension in arteries and blood vessels, helping to reduce blood pressure. It can help to prevent coronary heart disease and keep away many cardiovascular issues, including reducing the risk of heart disease in post menopausal women. Since it tends to thin the blood, it can help with preventing future blood clots, and also may help to stabilize cholesterol.

Women's Health Issues

Red clover is great for women's health problems, such as menopausal and menstrual issues. It can help to lessen the severity of menstrual cramps and can help to eliminate hot flashes and minimize bone loss.

Culinary

The flowers of the red clover taste good and have a slightly honey-like flavor. The greens can also be eaten raw in salads. In addition, dried red clover petals can replace up to 25% of the flour in any recipe of baked goods. The petals should be dried completely, and then pulverized in a food processor to as fine of a powder as possible.

Other Uses

Red clover can be used to support proper lymphatic function, to boost the immune system, to promote healthy skin, and to balance endocrine function. In addition to its medicinal uses, red clover has historically been, and is still used as an animal fodder.

Dosage:

        Tincture: 10-20 drops up to three times per day
        Tea: Up to three cups per day
        Poultice, Compress, Salve: As needed.
        Syrup: one teaspoon once or twice per day.

Some folklore about Red Clover:

-   To dream of a field of clovers is considered to be lucky.
-   If a woman is to place a leaf of a red clover in her shoe, then the first man she meets after that will be the man she will marry.
-   Usually the plant has three leaves, but can also have either two, four, or five. There is lore associated with each of these:

- o Two leaves – Place the leaf under your pillow to dream of your future lover.
- o Three leaves – Carry this leaf to detect witches, sorcerers, and fairies.
- o Four leaves – Carry for good luck, or to drive evil away.
- o Five leaves – Carried by witches to make them more powerful. Considered a very unlucky find.

Valerian (Valeriana officinalis)

Properties: Antispasmodic, Anxiolytic, Sedative, Nervine.

Common Uses: Sleep disorders, Restlessness, Nervous disorders.

Common Preparations: Tea, Pill

Contraindications: Do not mix with alcohol or sedatives. Do not take if pregnant or give to children under 3 years of age. Do not take if you have liver disease.

Plant parts used: Root

Possible Side Effects

Valerian is considered very safe, and usually, there are no side effects felt on waking when valerian is used as a sleep aid. In some occasions, side effects such as headache, stomachache, or dry mouth may be experienced by some.

Plant Identification

Valerian is native to Europe and Asia. It is a perennial plant which thrives even in harsh winter climates. When fully grown, the plant can stand up to five feet tall with dark green leaves in seven to ten leaflet pairs. Roots should be harvested in fall or in early spring and should be laid to dry outdoors because they tend to release an unpleasant smell as they dry out. The stems of the valerian plant are hollow. The flowers are very sweet and fragrant and can be white or pink. They should be harvested in early summer if they are to be used, or to prevent the spread of the plant.

Historical Uses

Valerian root has been used by health practitioners for hundreds of years for sleep issues and nervous disorders, and was commonly prescribed in ancient Greece, Rome, and in medieval Sweden.

Antispasmodic

May prevent sudden or involuntary muscle contractions. Valerian has been used to help to relieve the symptoms of Parkinson's disease, and also restless leg syndrome.

Anxiolytic/ Nervine

Valerian root tea has been shown to decrease nervousness and restlessness, as well as to relieve symptoms of anxiety and depression. The root can help to ease anxious feelings that arise due to stressful situations and may also help with chronic conditions characterized by anxious behaviors, like generalized anxiety disorder or OCD. The tea can help to increase focus and reduce hyperactive behavior in children. Valerian regulates the nerve impulses in brain and nervous system and can improve the response to stress by maintaining levels of serotonin.

Sedative

Often called "nature's valium," the most widely recognized use for valerian is to help with sleep disorders and improving sleep quality. Studies have shown that valerian root helps to improve insomnia symptoms in postmenopausal women when taken before bedtime. The sedative effects of valerian help people to fall asleep faster, stay asleep longer, and get a more restorative sleep. Some studies also suggest that it might be helpful for children with sleep problems as well, though it is best to seek the guidance of a health care practitioner for dosing information before giving to children.

Other Uses

The flowers of valerian have been used to make perfume for centuries and can also be used to help those suffering from withdrawal from benzodiazepines. Valerian has a similar effect on cats as does catnip.

Dosage:

Tea: As needed, before bed or during the day to relieve anxiety.

Tincture: Up to 20 drops

Pill: For anxiety, about 120 to 200 mg three times per day, as a sleep aid, 400 to 900 mg taken 30 minutes to two hours before bed.

Some folklore about Valerian:

- It was believed to have aphrodisiac qualities in medieval England, and it was said that if a lady carried valerian with her, she would never lack for suitors.
- Believed to increase psychic perception.
- It is said that the pied piper of Hamelin actually used valerian to lure the rats from Hamelin rather than his music.

Yarrow (Achillea millefolium)

Properties: Antibacterial, Antimicrobial, Anxiolytic, Astringent, Diuretic.

Common Uses: Fever, Colds, Hay fever, Menstruation issues, Diarrhea, Loss of appetite, Digestive issues, induce sweating, Toothache, Stop bleeding

Common Preparations: Tea, Poultice, Compress, Pills, Bath, Tincture

Contraindications: Do not use during pregnancy. Do not use in those with allergy to the Aster family of flowers. Do not use for children under 5 years old because of potential allergic reaction.

Part of Plant used: Above-ground parts (stems, leaves, flowers)

Possible Side Effects

Yarrow is considered safe for humans, though in rare cases may cause drowsiness and an increase in urination.

Plant Identification

Yarrow, also known as thousand leaf, woundwort, and the nosebleed plant, is related to the daisy plant, and consists of dark green, finely divided leaves, and flower clusters with small, flat, white, sometimes pink, flowers. The stalk can grow up to one meter tall and is a perennial which blooms from June to November. Other members of the Asteraceae family include chamomile, chrysanthemum, feverfew, and sunflower. Collect the flowers while flowering during the summer or early autumn. The leaves can be collected all year round.

Historical Uses

Food and medicinal uses of yarrow have been documented back to at least 1200 BCE, where in the story of the Trojan war, Achilles was said to have carried Yarrow when he entered battle so that he could treat the wounds of his fellow soldiers. Yarrow has also been called, historically, *herba militaris* for this reason, and was widely used for treating cuts, scrapes, and minor wounds obtained in battle. As a vegetable in the 17th century, the young leaves and flowers eaten in salad, and also cooked much the same way that spinach is used today.

Antibacterial / Antimicrobial

In emergencies, the raw yarrow leaves can be placed on wounds. The leaves should be bruised so that their juices come out, and then placed directly onto the wound to protect it until it can be properly cleaned out and dressed.

Anti-inflammatory

The anti-inflammatory properties of yarrow are often used as a compress for hemorrhoids or other swellings on the body.

Anxiolytic

The anti-anxiety effects of yarrow are particularly useful during times of chronic stress, and a tea or pill can be used to calm the nerves and clear the mind.

Astringent

A compress of yarrow is useful for toning varicose veins. The astringent properties also make it useful as a facial compress or added to face wash and shampoo. As a bath, yarrow can help to soothe irritated skin, clarify skin, and clear up chronic redness.

Bleeding and Blood disorders

One of the most well known uses for yarrow is its ability to stop bleeding and to move stagnant blood. It can help to prevent and clear blood clots and can also help to lower high blood pressure. A poultice of yarrow will help to heal a bruise or a blood blister faster and helps to improve circulation. As one of the alternate names of yarrow suggests, it is often used for stopping nosebleeds. For this purpose, a fresh yarrow leaf can be bruised, rolled up, and inserted into the affected nostril. Leave the leaf inserted until the bleeding stops.

Fevers

A hot tea of yarrow can be drunk to induce sweating and help to reduce a fever. It helps to relax the skin and open the pores to allow for sweating and the release of toxins. Taking yarrow bath or tea at the beginning of a cold or a fever will help to reduce the duration of the symptoms.

Diuretic

Tea or pills of yarrow can act as a diuretic, although care must be taken in those with chronic kidney diseases.

Women's Health

Drinking yarrow tea three times per day for three days can reduce menstrual pain and help to reduce heavy menstrual bleeding. It can normalize blood flow, calm heavy periods, and re-start suppressed periods.

Other Uses

Infusions of yarrow are used for cosmetic cleansers topically, such as face wash and used as a hair rinse. When applied topically, yarrow tea can also act as an insect repellent.

Dosage:

> Tea: One to three cups per day as needed
> Compress, Salve: Use as needed

Some folklore about Yarrow:

- Yarrow was used during the middle ages during exorcism, both because of its ability to summon the devil, and its ability to drive him away.
- Used by the druids for predicting the weather.

Chapter 4: Medicinal Preparations to Make With Your Herbs

In order to make full use of the benefits of herbs that are growing in your garden or gathered through foraging, they need to be prepared in the right way. Some herbs will be rendered ineffective if placed in boiling water, and others are not beneficial if taken internally. Most herbs are water soluble, but some work better when infused into alcohol. In the previous chapters, some notes were made regarding the proper ways to use the herbs that were discussed, and in this chapter more information will be given regarding how to make these preparations.

Some herbal preparations can be used internally, others must be used externally only, and there are also some preparations which can be used either internally or externally.

Teas, tinctures, pills, and syrups are most commonly used as the herbal equivalent to medications, taken on a regular schedule in order to provide relief for various health concerns. Salves, Poultices, Baths, and Compresses are used externally only, although preparing them is somewhat similar to preparing a tea. Oils can be used either internally or externally. Externally, they are used as massage oils, and can sometimes be used for culinary purposes as well.

One of the things to consider when choosing what sort of herbal preparation to use, is that the idea is to get the active ingredients from the herb as close to the affected area as possible. For example, if the problem is a sore throat, then a tea would be appropriate, whereas a tea may not be the best way if the issue is arthritis of the knee, where a compress may be more useful.

Some important notes about the preparations on the following pages:

A nonreactive pan is often called for, and indicates a pot or pan made from a material that will not react with the ingredients. Some of the herbs used may be acidic in nature, and there is a danger that the acids in the mixture may leach metals out of 'reactive pans' such as aluminum, cast iron, or copper. These types of pans or pots should not be used for creating herbal preparations. For the recipes that specify non-reactive, use stainless steel, ceramic, or glass for cooking.

Some of the preparations call for a tempered glass jar. Tempered glass is a type of glass that is prepared in a way that it can be safely heated without the risk of shattering. This is important when adding a hot preparation into a jar. Jars that are used for canning, like a mason jar is made from tempered glass. If no tempered glass is available, or if you are not sure what type of glass you have, then make sure to cool the liquid before adding it to the jar so that there is no danger that the glass will break.

Herbal Teas

Tea is probably the easiest way to prepare any herb and will be familiar to most people. We usually think of tea being made from dried leaves, but they can also be made using fresh. Note that not all herbs should be used fresh; generally, it is just the leaves that are used fresh and not the flowers or the roots. If in doubt, use the dried herb. Tea is relaxing before bed for those with trouble sleeping, helping to calm the mind and the body. For a person with respiratory issues, hot tea will deliver the needed herbal preparation, but the steam from the tea will also help to open swollen sinuses. Teas often have quick results since they are quickly absorbed by the body.

A tea is an infusion or a decoction that extracts the water soluble components from a plant. Teas made with the leaves, flowers, and other softer parts of the plant are made by infusion, where the herbs are steeped in water that has been boiled. The harder parts of the plant such as the roots, berries, or bark, need to be processed a little more in order to extract the active

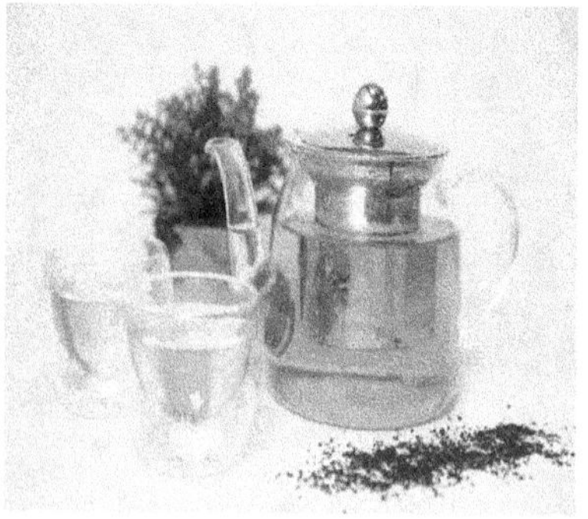

ingredients, so they are boiled along with the water. Instructions for both methods are included below.

Best herbs for herbal tea:

- Burdock
- Calendula
- Chickweed
- Dandelion
- Echinacea
- Elder
- Marshmallow
- Mullein
- Nettle
- Peppermint
- Plantain
- Red Clover
- Valerian
- Yarrow

When to use an herbal tea:

Tea is warming, soothing, and calming. It is the ideal preparation to use for any issues with the throat or digestive issues. It is especially well suited for issues where the warming effect and the steam can work with the herbs to provide a sense of relaxation, such as when suffering from a cold or flu, or before bed. Because of the relaxing qualities of a hot cup of tea, it is also ideal for nervous disorders and stress.

Equipment:

- Kettle or saucepan to boil water (for an infusion)
- Saucepan (for a decoction)
- Mug
- Strainer or cheesecloth to strain the herbs, or a tea ball to contain the loose herbs

Components:

- Water
- Dried herbs (or fresh leaves)
    - A general rule of thumb is to use two to four tablespoons of a dried herb for each cup of water used. This amount may need to be adjusted for taste.
    - For fresh herbs, use double the amount of herb (¼ to ½ cup)

Infusion Method:

To make a perfect cup of herbal tea, use a handful of fresh leaves or about a tablespoon of dried herbs for every cup of water. The flavor or strength of the tea can be adjusted to your taste. If using fresh leaves, then coarsely chop them before adding to the water.

Place the herbs into a cup or pot and add boiling water. If using dry herbs, they can be placed into a tea ball, or there are also several disposable and reusable teabag-like products that can be purchased for making loose leaf tea. Another good way to make an infusion is to use a French press, which will strain the herbs. Steep for 10 minutes, until the tea has acquired the desired strength. Determining the desired strength may take some practice, but a good rule of thumb is to steep for 10 minutes. If you find that the tea was too strong, steep for less time next time, if you feel that it was not strong enough, then steep for longer. Strain the tea if needed and serve hot, adding lemon or honey to taste. One special note is that due to the stinging needles on nettle, it is not recommended to use the infusion method for fresh herbs, but instead to follow the decoction method.

Cold teas have the same benefits as hot teas and may be preferable during the summer. To make a cold infusion, place the herbs into a mason jar with a lid and cover with cold water and place in the refrigerator. A cold infusion will need to steep for quite a lot longer than a hot infusion and is typically steeped overnight for use the next day.

Decoction Method:

A decoction is used when the components are more difficult to extract, as in woody stems, bark, or roots. In a pot, heat water, and the herbs until boiling, and then reduce the heat and simmer for 30 minutes. Strain the tea into a cup and enjoy.

Again, the strength of the tea may be adjusted according to taste.

How do I make a tea using one ingredient that requires infusion and one that requires decoction?

The best way to handle this is to make the decoction first, and then use the water from the decoction to steep the herbs that should be infused.

Some useful herb mixtures for tea:

1. Immune Boosting Tea – Echinacea infusion and Elderberry syrup.

Prepare an infusion from ¼ cup of dried echinacea flowers in one cup of water. Once the infusion has steeped, add elderberry syrup to taste.

This tea should be taken at the first signs of a cold or flu to boost immunity and shorten the duration of symptoms. Take one cup of tea three times per day for two days.

2. Fever Relief Tea – Yarrow, Peppermint, and Elderflower infusion.

Prepare an infusion with one tablespoon of dried yarrow, one tablespoon of dried peppermint, and one tablespoon of dried elderflowers in one cup of water. Honey may be added to taste if desired.

This tea should be taken to encourage sweating in those with high fevers and is also relaxing for those suffering from a cold or flu.

3. Antioxidant and Antiinflammatory Tea – Red clover, Nettle, and Peppermint infusion

Prepare an infusion with two tablespoons of dried nettle leaves, one tablespoon of peppermint leaves, and one tablespoon of red clover flowers in one cup of water.

The nettle provides strong antiinflammatory properties, and the clover and peppermint are antioxidants.

> 4. Tonic Tea for cold weather – Nettle, Peppermint, Mullein, Dandelion, Red Clover

Prepare an infusion with four teaspoons of dried nettle leaves, three teaspoons of peppermint, two teaspoons of mullein, and two teaspoons of dandelion leaf. Let it steep for 15 minutes in 1 cup of boiled water and then strain well.

This tea is very warming and soothing to the body during the cold months of the year.

Of course, there are several herbs that make a great tea on their own:

1. Yarrow tea for colds and fevers.
2. Burdock root tea to lower blood pressure and help heal a damaged liver.
3. Mullein tea for chronic cough and asthma.
4. Dandelion root tea to help eliminate toxins and help the immune system fight infections.

Syrups

Syrups are prepared with dried herbs and sugar or honey and are a good way to preserve herbs. It is also a good way to get the benefit from herbs that may not taste that great since the result will be quite sweet regardless of the herb used. Generally, to make a syrup, an herbal infusion or tea is mixed in equal amounts with honey or sugar. One of the benefits of syrups are that they are able to stick to and to coat membranes and are particularly useful for calming coughs.

The best herbs for syrups:

- Elder
- Marshmallow
- Mullein
- Red Clover

Reasons for using a syrup:

Syrups can be used as a sweetener in teas or other drinks or can be used as an ingredient in cooking or cocktail making. The texture of a syrup, as well as the honey, make it very soothing to a sore throat or as a cough syrup.

Equipment:

- Non-reactive saucepan with a lid
- Bottle or jar with a lid for the finished syrup

Components:

- One cup of herbal infusion or decoction
- One cup of honey or sugar

Method:

With the desired herb(s), create an infusion or decoction. Typically, the infusion or decoction is made about twice as strong (using twice as many herbs) than would be used for a tea. You will need to have a total of one cup of herbal infusion and/or decoction. Once the infusion and/or decoction is prepared, place it on the stove and add one cup of honey or sugar and warm until combined, without boiling.

Take the mixture off the stove and let it cool completely before bottling. Store the finished syrup in a bottle or jar in a dark place or in the refrigerator for up to six months.

For making a syrup, either honey or sugar can be used. The goal is to have an equal amount of strong tea and sweetener, about one cup of each. If the syrup is made 1:1 as in the above recipe, then it will be shelf stable and can be stored in a dark, cool place. If a different consistency is desired, either a thinner syrup or less sweetness, then a syrup can also be made with two parts of water to one part honey or even three parts tea to one part honey. However, if less honey is used, then the syrup will need to be kept in the refrigerator.

If desired, a little bit of tincture can be added to the syrup to prolong the shelf life slightly or to add the properties of an additional herb. The tincture should be added right before the syrup is placed in the bottle, after it has been removed from the heat.

Cough Syrup with Mullein and Elderflower

First, prepare an infusion of two tablespoons mullein flowers, one tablespoon mullein leaves, and one tablespoon elderflowers. Steep this mixture in one cup of boiling water for 10 minutes, then strain. Place the infusion on low heat and add one cup of honey, stirring until the honey is dissolved. Store in the refrigerator for up to three months and take a dose of one teaspoon every three to four hours as needed for congestion and cough.

Of course, there are several herbs that make a great medicinal syrup on their own:

1. Elderberry syrup for colds, flu, and immune boosting
2. Red clover syrup for lymphatic congestion
3. Peppermint syrup for indigestion

Culinary herbal simple syrups:

For culinary use, a syrup is generally made with sugar instead of honey, but either can be used. The syrups are made by combining one cup of an infusion with one cup of white sugar, heated until the sugar is dissolved. These syrups can be used to make a sorbet, for making cakes or deserts, use to sweeten iced tea or lemonade, mix with sparkling water for homemade soda, use to flavor cocktails. Popular flavors include Peppermint and Elderflower.

Herbal Oils

Herbal oils are different from essential oils. The essential oils are oils produced by the plant, and usually extracted by cold pressing or steam. Herbal oils are oils, usually inert nut oils, infused with herbs.

The best herbs for making herbal oils:

- Burdock
- Calendula
- Chickweed
- Marshmallow
- Mullein

Reasons to use herbal oil:

An herbal oil is needed as an ingredient for making a salve, but also can be used directly on the skin as a massage oil. Applying herbal oils to the skin can help to calm some skin issues and can be absorbed by the skin to help with muscular and joint problems as well. Be sure to choose your base oil and herb according to the desired outcome. These herbal oils are not meant to be taken internally.

Equipment:

- A jar with a tight-fitting lid

Components:

-   Enough herb to fill the selected jar.
-   Enough oil to fill the jar to the top

Methods:

There are two main ways to make herbal oils, either the windowsill method, which takes several weeks, or the stovetop method, which takes approximately an hour. Most herbalists will prefer the windowsill method because it is gentler to the herbs and can extract more of the useful properties from the dried herbs. The stovetop method also works, but may result in the herbal oil being less potent.

Windowsill Method: Dry the herbs completely before making oil. Place the desired herb in a clean jar with a tight-fitting lid, labeling it and packing with about one inch of space above the herbs, so there is space for the oil. Add oil to the jar, making sure to completely cover the herbs. Cap tightly and shake well. Leave the jar in a sunny window and shake one to two times per day for up to two weeks. Strain the oil into a clean, dry jar, label, and store it in a cool dark place.

Stovetop Method: Place herbs and oil into a double boiler. Bring water in the bottom of the double boiler to a boil, then simmer over very low heat for 30-60 minutes. Keep the lid on so that the essential oils do not escape. Generally, to make one cup of oil, you will need one cup of your chosen oil and two cups of dried herb. Using the stovetop method is much quicker, but the oil produced is not quite as high quality and will not absorb as much of the qualities of the herb as the windowsill method will.

Various oils can be used, or a blend of oils. Usually almond, jojoba, or grapeseed are oils that are used because they are fairly inert (plain with very little smell) and because they are nourishing oils for using on the skin for topical applications.

The final color of the oil may vary depending on the herbs added. For example, a calendula oil would be golden in color, whereas a mint oil would be darker, or even a light green. The color may also vary depending on the base oil used.

Dried herbs must be used for this preparation because any water or moisture from the plants will add to the risk of the herbal oil growing mold or bacteria while infusing, or while it is in storage. In order to dry the herbs, spread them on a drying rack out of direct sunlight. Usually, they will be completely dry within 3-5 days but may take longer depending on humidity and other factors. A food dehydrator may be used as well.

Choosing the base oil to use:

You want something that is going to have a decent shelf life, and that is odorless since you want the properties of the herb to be the main focus, not the carrier oil. You would also want something vicious, especially if it will be used for massage.

Grapeseed: Astringent, toning, emollient. Nonallergenic, good for sensitive skin. Shelf life 3-4 months

Sweet almond: High in vitamin E, protective and nourishing.   Good for all skin types, especially used for babies. Stable shelf life

Jojoba: Very thick oil, especially used for acne control, antiinflammatory properties, and useful for sunburns.

Olive: Useful for repair of damaged or dry skin, soothing to inflammatory skin conditions, stable shelf life, antiinflammatory, antioxidant

Do not use mineral oil, soybean, corn, peanut, or palm oil. These oils can prevent the absorption of the herb and may also present problems of allergic reaction.

If there is any change in color or smell of the oil over time, then it should be discarded.

Here are a few good options for herbal oils:

Mullein oil:

-   Antiseptic, good for relieving congestion when rubbed on the chest, astringent, mucolytic.

-   Used for hemorrhoids, wound healing, nerve pain

Chickweed Oil:

-   Used for hot or inflamed skin, and for joint conditions.
-   Toning astringent for diaper rash and childhood eczema

Calendula Oil:

-   Antiinflammatory, astringent.
-   Healing wounds, rashes, abrasions, eczema, psoriasis, fungal infections, acne.

Salves

A salve is a solid, which is a combination of oils and wax. Beeswax is traditionally used, but a good vegan option may be soy wax or cocoa butter. Salve works a little like lotion. It often will be a solid oil, which melts in the hands and is then massaged into the skin.

The best herbs for salves:

- Aloe
- Calendula
- Chickweed
- Marshmallow
- Nettle
- Mullein
- Oats
- Plantain

Reasons to use a salve:

Salve can be used in any area and is especially useful when massaged into skin to soften dry skin or soothe sore muscles. It can also be used to promote healing of scars, and ease neuralgia (nerve pain). By adding beeswax to the salve, you are also adding the softening, soothing, antioxidant, anti-inflammatory, antibacterial, and antiallergenic properties to the finished salve.

Equipment:

- Double boiler
- Container for salve

Components:

- One cup of herbal oil
- ¼ cup of beeswax

Method:

In order to make a salve, the first step is to make an herbal oil using any of the methods described in the previous section. You will need one cup of oil for one batch of salve.

Place ¼ cup of beeswax shavings or beeswax beads in a double boiler on low heat. Once the beeswax has melted, remove the pan from the heat and stir in the herbal oil. The salve should be placed into containers while hot and then left to sit and harden at room temperature.

If you want a harder salve – more like a solid massage bar, then use more beeswax. For a more lotion-type consistency use less beeswax. Finding the ideal consistency may take some experimentation. The salve should be stored in a cool, dry place, or in the refrigerator. If the salve becomes too liquid, then it can be placed into the refrigerator to harden up. If it becomes hard, then it will usually soften with body heat.

It is important not to let any water get into the salve, as this can promote the growth of mold and bacteria. If not refrigerated, the shelf life of the sale is about six months. If refrigerated, it will last for up to one year.

To make a vegan salve (without beeswax), cocoa butter or a soy wax can be used for the beeswax in the recipe.

To store salves, wide mouthed jam jars or metal tins are perfect containers, or anything that has a tight lid. Another option is to use a twist-up container such as a lipstick container to make a lip salve, or a deodorant container to make a twist-up massage stick, which can be applied directly to the skin without handling it. Many different types of containers are available for purchase online quite cheaply.

One herb that is used differently to the recipe above is aloe vera. Aloe vera does not need to be infused in oil since it is already a gel and can just be mixed with olive oil before adding to the beeswax. To make one cup of this mixture, use about ½ cup each of aloe vera gel and olive oil and mix well.

Here are some useful salve recipes:
Burdock root and leaf plus mullein leaf.
This will create an all-purpose salve which can be used anywhere on the body.
Red clover salve.

This salve works to care for chapped lips and itchy dry skin.

Yarrow salve.

Used for hemorrhoids, bruises, and varicose veins.

Plantain and Dandelion leaf

Stings and bites and soothes itchy skin.

Tinctures

A tincture is a preparation that is made by steeping leaves, flowers, bark, roots, or seeds in an alcohol solution. The result is more potent than a tea, and generally only a few drops are taken at a time. Herbs that are prepared this way have a long shelf life and are more convenient to use than many other preparations.

Best herbs for tinctures:

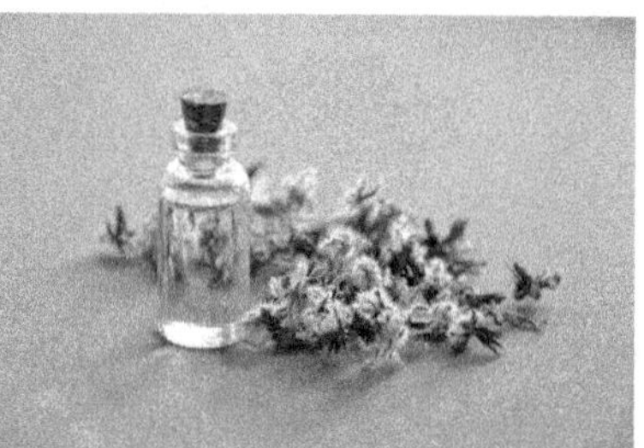

- Burdock
- Calendula
- Chickweed
- Echinacea
- Elder
- Marshmallow
- Mullein
- Nettle
- Red Clover
- Yarrow

Reasons to use a tincture:

Having a tincture is quite convenient because only a few drops or a dropper full is needed. In addition, many herbs are more easily absorbed into the body via alcohol rather than water. Also, some of the active components may not be water-soluble, and so may only be available when absorbed through alcohol.

Equipment needed:

- Knife
- Airtight jar or mason jar for steeping
- Dark glass bottle(s) with a dropper for finished product
- Cheesecloth for straining

Components:

- Fresh or dried herbs
- Alcohol (at least 80 proof) such as vodka or brandy. The bottle should say 40% alcohol by volume or higher.

Method:

If using fresh herbs, then you will need equal amounts of alcohol to chopped herbs. If using dried herbs, then you will need approximately four times as much alcohol as chopped herb.

Place the herbs and the alcohol in an airtight jar and place it aside for six weeks to give time for the alcohol to absorb all of the components of the herb. The jar should be shaken a few times per week, but not opened during this time.

After the herbs have infused in the alcohol, open the jar and strain the liquid into a labeled container with a dropper for easier dosing.

This procedure can also be used to make herbal vinegars for those who do not wish to consume alcohol. Simply add apple cider vinegar in place of the alcohol.

Here are a few suggestions for useful herbal tinctures:

Mullein tincture for colds and respiratory problems.

Elderberry tincture to reduce inflammation.

Echinacea tincture to boost immune system.

Herbal Pills

There are three types of herbal preparations that are designed for ingesting, capsules, pills, or lozenges. The type that is used is depending on the herb and your preference. Since this type of preparation is usually meant for more long-term use, and is much more concentrated than taking a tea, it is best to consult an herbalist or other professional before making herbal pills the main part of your herbal remedy regime.

Pills are most effective when made with bark, root, or seeds. Pills made with leaves or flowers will not have as long of a shelf life.

Best herbs for herbal pills:

- Burdock
- Calendula
- Dandelion
- Marshmallow
- Peppermint
- Valerian
- Yarrow

Reasons for taking herbal pills:

Some teas are not pleasant tasting, and in addition, there are some ailments for which it might be more convenient to take a pill instead of brewing teas. The pills are more time consuming to make but have a fairly long shelf life so a supply can be made ahead of time. Additionally, if several herbal preparations are to be taken, they might not mix well in a single tea, but the components can be added to a capsule or a pill for convenience.

Equipment needed:

- Blender or food processor
- Gelatin capsules (optional)

Components:

- Two cups of finely powdered herb or herb mixture
- Up to one cup of honey or water, only use the minimum amount needed to create a paste.

Method:

Pills are made by creating a paste from powdered dry herb by adding a little honey or water until the mixture is about the consistency of bread dough. The paste can be rolled into ropes and then cut into small segments to make small balls that are about the size of peas. They should not be too big as they are designed to be swallowed whole, and there should not be a choking hazard. Pills can be rolled in powdered marshmallow root to prevent them from sticking to each other, and once they are all made, lay them on a baking sheet covered with parchment and bake them for about 2-3 hours at the lowest oven temperature, then place them somewhere where they can continue to dry. Pills may take a few days to dry if made with honey instead of water.

Two cups of herb to one cup of honey or water should yield about 50 pills. These can last one to two years if kept in an airtight container, but do not use if you notice any change in color or smell.

Lozenges are made in the same way as a pill but can be a bit larger as they are designed to be sucked rather than swallowed. This can be used for herbs that are more pleasant tasting and are particularly helpful for herbs that can help to relieve pain or inflammation in the throat, such as marshmallow.

Capsules are made by drying and powdering the herb or mixture of herbs that is to be used, and then measuring the powdered herb into a gelatin capsule. Gelatin capsules can be purchased online or from some pharmacies or herbal shops. Some retailers also carry vegan gelatin capsules. Once the capsule is filled, close it with the other half of the capsule, and then store in an airtight container in a cool dry place. If you need to make a lot of capsules, there are machines on the market to help you fill and cap the capsules as it can be quite time consuming to create each capsule separately by hand. There are different sizes of capsules available, and each will hold a different dose of herb. In general, a size 'ooo' capsule will hold 1000 mg of powder, which equals 1 gram. However, these capsules are quite large and may be difficult to swallow.

Here are a few herbal mixtures that would work well in pill form. Each of them contains two different herbs, so use one cup of each powdered herb for the preparation.

A pill to soothe digestion: Marshmallow root + yarrow

A cough lozenge: Marshmallow root + burdock root

A capsule to help with sleep: Valerian root + oat

Baths

A bath is prepared in a similar way to a tea, but larger as it is for a tub instead of a teacup. A bath is a great way to use herbs that have positive effects on the skin or when larger areas are affected.

Best herbs for herbal baths:

- Calendula
- Dandelion
- Elder
- Oats
- Plantain
- Yarrow

Reasons for using an herbal bath:

Baths are a great way to relieve aching muscles and soothe joints, but they also do wonders for mental health as well. Having a warm bath when suffering from a cold will relax the whole body, relieve tension, and stimulate circulation. A bath is also great for encouraging digestion; it can soften the skin, clear or calm skin irritations like eczema and psoriasis, and also aids in a restful sleep.

Equipment needed:

- Cheesecloth or clean linen or cotton fabric.

Components:

- About ½ cup to one cup of dried herb.

Method:

The drawback of adding herbs directly to the bath is that the cleanup can be messy. In order to prevent cleanup, place the herbs into a square of clean cotton, linen, or cheesecloth and tie together to make a bundle. Drop the bundle into the water while the bath is filling up and allow to steep in the warm bath water while you bathe. The bundle itself may also be used as a washcloth to spread the active ingredients over the affected areas. This works especially well if using oats.

Another method is to make a pot of very strong herbal tea, steeping up to one cup of herb into four cups of water for about 20 minutes, and then straining the liquid and adding the strained tea to the bath.

Either of these methods will reduce the amount of cleanup needed without compromising the effectiveness of the herbs.

To add detoxification, muscle relaxant, and skin softening properties to any herbal bath, ½ cup of either sea salt or Epsom salt can be added to the infusion or added to the bath tea bundle.

The herbs listed above can each be used alone, mixed with a salt, or used in one of the following recipes for added benefit:

Calendula and Rose to soften skin

Mix ½ cup of dried calendula petals and ¼ cup of dried rose petals with ½ cup of sea salt or Epsom salt. Add all of these ingredients to a square of fabric and tie together before adding to the bath. Before getting into the bath, ½ cup of jojoba or almond oil can also be added to the bathwater for an extra soothing bath.

Chickweed and Vinegar for itchy skin

In a blender, mix two tablespoons of apple cider vinegar with ½ cup of fresh chickweed until it is all combined and smooth. More vinegar or a little water can be added if needed to make the mixture smooth. Strain through a cheesecloth, and then add to a warm bath to relieve itchy skin.

Dandelion and Violet Bath for removing toxins

Wash and chop about 1 ½ to two cups each of fresh dandelion and violets. Both leaves and flowers can be used from both plants. Place them in a bowl and cover with four cups of water and steep for 20 minutes. Strain the liquid into a warm bath. If desired, tie up the flowers and leaves that were used to create the infusion and add that to the bath as well.

Oatmeal Bath to soothe skin

Tie one cup of rolled oats (not instant oatmeal) into a cloth and add to the bath while the water is running. While bathing, rub the bundle gently on the skin in any areas that are dry or irritated. This bath is especially good for kids with eczema or psoriasis.

Elderflower and Milk Bath for softening and soothing skin

In a clean piece of cloth, add six fresh elderflower clusters, or two tablespoons of dried flowers, with ¼ cup of dried milk powder and add to a warm, not hot, bath.

Poultices

A poultice is a method where a paste made from fresh or dried herbs is spread on the affected part of the body and covered with a warm cloth. Usually they are used to relieve inflammation and to promote healing. The warmth of the poultice increases blood flow to the affected area.

Poultices work best if they are kept warm and moist. In order to retain the warmth and moisture, the area can be wrapped with plastic wrap, or a hot water bottle or heating pad can be placed over top of the cloths or bandages holding the poultice to the skin.

The poultice should be removed before it gets cold, but a new one can be applied if needed.

Once the poultice is removed, the area should be washed with water, or a calendula infusion. Applying the poultice may be repeated daily until the condition has resolved.

Best herbs to use for a poultice:

- Burdock
- Chickweed
- Dandelion
- Elder
- Mullein
- Red Clover

- Plantain
- Yarrow

Reasons for using a poultice:

A hot poultice is a great way to treat respiratory conditions such as pneumonia, bronchitis, and congestion. It can also help to stimulate circulation, improve organ function, reduce inflammation. It is a good way to treat infection and to draw infection out of the body.

Caution must be used to check for allergic reaction since the herb is in very close contact with the skin.

The amount of herb used will depend on the size of the area to be treated. The goal is to have a very thick paste completely covering the affected area, and the cloth should be large enough to cover the entire poultice in order to prevent it from falling away. A small amount of poultice may also be held in place with an adhesive bandage.

Fresh herbs tend to work better than dried and have a stronger effect on the affected area. However, using dried herbs a poultice is easier to make, and less messy. Dried leaves or petals, powdered roots, bark, or berries work well with this method.

To prepare the skin for a poultice, the affected area should be clean and clear of any debris or dirt. The skin can be cleaned with a calendula tea or tincture to ensure that the area is clean. If there is danger of an allergic reaction, then it may also be a good idea to cover the skin with a thin layer of oil before applying the poultice. Grapeseed, olive, or almond oil will work well for this purpose. The healing benefits of the herb will still enter the skin through the oil, but it may reduce the allergic reaction. If an allergic reaction is noticeable, such as itching or redness, the poultice should be removed, and the area washed thoroughly with soap and water.

Equipment needed to make a poultice:

- Cotton or linen cloth to cover the poultice
- Bandage or a length of fabric to attach the cloth to the body
- Mortar and pestle

Components:

- Fresh or dried herbs
- Hot water, or herbal tea as needed

Method:

For fresh herbs, roughly chop them and then mash with a mortar and pestle, adding hot water or herbal tea in small amounts until a thick paste is made.

Another method for using fresh leaves is to blanch them by cooking them for about 1 minute in boiling water and then plunging them in ice to halt the cooking process. The blanched leaves can then be placed directly on the skin and covered with a clean cloth.

For dried herbs, add the herbs to a mortar and crush them with a pestle, adding enough hot water or herbal tea to make a rough paste. Apply to the skin and cover with a cloth.

An emergency poultice can also be used in a situation where the herb is available, but there is no time or equipment available to make a proper poultice. This could be useful while camping or out in the woods in the case of an insect bite, a scrape, or a splinter.

If the fresh herb is available, for example, yarrow, plantain, or mullein leaf, rinse it in water to remove any dirt or debris, and then crush the leaf/leaves between your fingers until the leaf is bruised and the juices begin to come out. Place the leaf/leaves on the area to be treated and cover it with a bandage or clean cloth for a few hours. This process can be repeated with new leaves if desired.

Compress

A compress is prepared similarly to a tea, as an infusion or decoction, though typically is about twice as strong. The mixture is then soaked into a clean cloth of cotton or linen and applied to the skin. The compress can be applied either warm or cool, and the cloth can be dipped back in the liquid to bring the liquid back to temperature.

Best herbs to use for a compress:

- Burdock
- Calendula
- Chickweed
- Dandelion
- Elder
- Mullein
- Peppermint
- Plantain
- Red Clover
- Yarrow

Reasons for using a compress:

A compress is used for skin issues, wounds, inflammations of the skin, arthritis (inflammation of the joints), headache

When to use hot and when to use cold:

Hot is used for relaxing, and cold is used for easing inflammation. In general, hot compress will ease muscle tension and arthritis, muscle spasms, menstrual pain. Cold compresses will relieve burns, headaches, ease pain. Cold will also constrict blood vessels, so can help to limit bruising.

Equipment needed to make a compress:

- Non-reactive pan if using a hot compress
- Bowl kept in the fridge for a cold compress
- Clean linen or cotton cloth

Components:

- Cheesecloth
- Herb to be used for the infusion or the decoction – general rule of thumb is to use approximately twice as much as would be used for a tea of the same herb.

Hot Compress Method:

- Bring about 4 cups of water to boil in a non-reactive pot.
- Reduce to a simmer and add about 1 cup of chopped herbs.
- For an infusion,

Cold Compress Method:

- Create an infusion or decoction with the desired herb(s)
- Steep the herbs in hot water for 20 minutes, and then strain through cheesecloth and place the mixture into the refrigerator until cool.
- Once the liquid has cooled down, dip the cloth into the mixture, wring out, and apply to the affected area for at least 10 minutes. The cloth may be re-dipped into the liquid if it warms up while sitting on the body.

Another type of compress is used in a Thai herbal compress massage, or Herbal Ball Compress Massage. In this type of treatment, which is used to relieve pain and inflammation, instead of making an infusion or decoction from the herbs, the herbs are wrapped into a ball.

About ½ cup of dried herb and ½ cup of rice powder is placed on a large square of clean cotton or linen fabric that is folded into quarters to add extra layers of fabric so that the herbs don't come out. Once the herbs are in place, gather the four corners and secure with some string. You should have a fairly solid ball of herbs. The compress can be used as is, or the ends of the fabric can be rolled up and tied with string to create a handle.

In a steamer pot, bring water to a boil, and place the herb ball in the steamer (not touching the water) for about 30-45 minutes.

After making sure that the ball is not too hot, place it on the affected area for up to 30 minutes.

Chapter 5: Culinary Uses of Common Herbs

While most herbs can be taken internally, some are more commonly used than others. Here are some recipes that you can use to use up some of the excess herbs in your garden. Don't forget that in cooking these herbs, they may lose some of their medicinal value, but will still retain their nutritional value. Many herbs are quite high in vitamins and minerals, especially vitamins C and K, and magnesium.

Burdock and Carrot Stir Fry

Often eaten in Asian cultures, the flavor and texture of the burdock root pairs wonderfully with that of carrots. This dish can be served warm or cold as a side dish with toasted sesame seeds on top.

Peel three to four gobo (burdock roots) and slice into two inch pieces. You should have about four cups of chopped and peeled root. Peel a large carrot and slice into two inch pieces. Cut the burdock root and the carrot into thin matchstick slices and then soak them in a bowl of cold water for 20 minutes. Heat about 1 ½ tablespoons of sesame oil in a large pan. Drain the burdock and carrot and then add to the pan over medium heat and stir fry for five to eight minutes. Add two tablespoons of sugar and a pinch of cayenne pepper and mix well. Add ¼ cup of soy sauce and continue to stir fry until the liquid has been absorbed. Sprinkle with toasted sesame seeds.

Calendula Scones

The bright and somewhat citrusy flavor of calendula petals lends itself very well to scones that can be served for an accompaniment to a spring brunch or picnic.

Combine two cups of all-purpose flour, ¼ cup sugar, one teaspoon of baking powder, and ¼ teaspoon of salt in a bowl and stir to mix. Add the zest of one lemon, ¼ cup of dried calendula blossoms, and ½ cup of cold cubed butter. Beat until the mixture is crumbly. Add ¼ cup lemon juice, ¼ cup of heavy cream, and one teaspoon vanilla extract. Beat until the mixture just starts to come together. Place on a floured surface and knead several times to create a smooth ball. Pat into a round disk about ½ inch thick, and score into six wedges with a knife. Sprinkle with coarse sugar and one teaspoon of calendula blossoms. Bake for 25 minutes at 350 degrees, then remove from the oven and cut through the disk at the score marks. Bake for five more minutes. Serve with butter and honey.

Chickweed Pesto

Since chickweed won't last very long once picked, if you have too much of it, then make a batch of this pesto, and it can be frozen until needed. Use it as part of a pasta sauce, add to scrambled eggs, or use as a sandwich filling.

To make the pesto, you will need about six-packed cups of freshly picked and washed chickweed, about 10 cloves of garlic, one cup of olive oil, one tablespoon of sea salt, and one cup of toasted walnuts. Add all ingredients in batches to a food processor and blend until smooth.

Dandelion With Lemon and Garlic

Dandelion is often overlooked as a green vegetable, but it cooks up nicely without losing a lot of its shape or texture. Just be sure to harvest away from sources of pollution because dandelion tends to retain toxins in its leaves.

You will need about 1½ pounds of dandelion leaves that have been washed and coarsely chopped. Heat two tablespoons of oil in a saute pan and add three cloves of garlic and a pinch of red pepper flakes. Cook until the garlic is browned, stirring frequently. Add the dandelion leaves with salt and pepper to taste. Saute for about 5 minutes, then remove from the heat and stir in the juice of one small lemon.

Elder Berry Muffins

Not a lot of people will have tasted elderberries before since they are not widely available commercially. The berries are small and can be quite tart. They do not have the same level of sweetness as blueberries or strawberries. Adding sugar and applesauce to this muffin recipe helps to even out the tartness, but the muffins can also be served with honey if they are still found to be too tart.

Combine two cups of flour, three teaspoons of baking powder, one teaspoon of salt, ¼ cup of sugar. Beat together one egg, ¼ cup applesauce, and one cup of milk. Mix the wet and dry ingredients and then stir in one cup of fresh or frozen elderberries. Fill muffin tins and bake at 425 degrees for 15-20 minutes.

Marshmallow Soup

A green vegetable may not be the first thing that comes to mind when thinking of marshmallow, but it makes a very nice thick soup when added at the end of the cooking process. Don't add the marshmallow leaves with the rest of the vegetables, or the mucilage will thicken the soup too much.

In a large pot, saute one diced onion, and then add one diced tomato, two diced bell peppers, six stalks of celery, diced. Dice and add four carrots, three large potatoes, and three cloves of garlic. Once the vegetables have started to brown, add six cups of chicken or vegetable stock and salt and pepper to taste. Simmer for 15-20 minutes, and then blend the soup with an immersion blender if desired. Chop two large handfuls of marshmallow leaves into ribbons fincly. Cook for 5 more minutes. Serve topped with croutons and chopped parsley.

Nettle Soup

Nettles can be intimidating to cook with because they are difficult to harvest and can cause quite a nasty rash if handled raw. Once the nettles are cooked, their stinging properties are lost, and they are safe to eat and to handle.

Using gloves, place six cups of nettles in a large pot of boiling salted water and boil for two minutes. Once done, place them in a bowl of ice water to stop the cooking process, then strain and set aside. Saute ½ cup shallots and ½ cup celery in olive oil until softened. Add one pound of baby potatoes, four cups of chicken stock, and one bay leaf. Simmer for five minutes. Add the nettles and enough water to cover the nettles and potatoes. Simmer for 15 minutes. Remove the bay leaf, take the soup off the heat, and puree the soup with an immersion blender. Add salt to taste, one tablespoon of lemon juice, and two to three tablespoons of heavy whipping cream.

Oat Pancakes

These pancakes are wonderfully fluffy and filling for breakfast on the weekend or make a large batch and warm them up in the toaster for quick breakfasts during the week.

Combine 1 ½ cups hulled oats with two cups of milk and let stand for five minutes. In another bowl, combine ½ cup whole wheat flour and ½ cup all-purpose flour with one tablespoon brown sugar, one tablespoon baking powder, ½ teaspoon salt, and ½ teaspoon cinnamon. Whisk two eggs and ¼ cup melted butter into the milk and oat mixture. Pour into flour mixture and stir until just combined. Bake about ¼ cup of batter per pancake on a skillet for about two minutes per side until golden.

Peppermint Watermelon Salad

There are no set measurements for this salad. All items can be added to taste, or according to what you have on hand. The combination makes a perfectly sweet and cooling salad for a picnic in the summer.

Fill a salad bowl with cubed watermelon and feta cheese. Sprinkle with sea salt, chopped peppermint, and basil leaves. Toss to combine. Optionally, you can sprinkle a little bit of a balsamic reduction over the top if desired.

Plantain and Egg Skillet

Plantain is another overlooked green that grows all over the place without really being noticed by people. The leaves of plantain cook and taste somewhat like spinach. The smaller new growth leaves taste great raw in a salad, but larger leaves can be a little bit tougher and do require cooking. The flower/seed stalk can be eaten too. It is best when lightly sautéed in butter or oil and tastes a little like asparagus.

Heat three tablespoons of olive oil in a skillet and add one diced onion. Cook until transparent, about five minutes. Add one pound of plantain leaves that have been washed and chopped. Season with salt and pepper. Stir gently while cooking until the leaves begin to wilt. Make four wells in the plantain mixture and crack one egg into each well. Cook for about four minutes longer, or until the eggs are set. Sprinkle with salt and pepper to taste.

Chapter 6: Your Herbal Medicine Cabinet

Most people, when they first learn about how herbs can help them in their everyday life get overwhelmed by all of the information that they gather on the herbs. In order to prevent information overload, it is best to focus on just a few preparations that will be used frequently. Listed below are all the herbs from this book, along with their most common uses.

Aloe vera	Burns and minor skin irritations
Burdock root	Lower blood pressure, relieve osteoarthritis
Calendula	Pain reducer, antiinflammatory
Chickweed	Constipation and bowel problems
Dandelion	Boost immune system
Echinacea	Help fight colds and flu

Elder	Relieve pain and heal bruises
Marshmallow	Reducing swelling
Mullein	Lung issues
Nettle	Reduce inflammation
Oats	Improve heart health
Peppermint	Digestive issues
Plantain	Reduce swelling
Red Clover	Women's issues
Valerian	Sleep disorders
Yarrow	Reduce fever

Incorporating herbs into your daily life will not happen overnight. It is best to focus on one or two herbs, or one or two issues that you wish to resolve and then go from there. Soon, the herbal knowledge will become second nature. For example, if you are suffering from arthritis, consider planting calendula, marshmallow, plantain, or nettle. If your family also suffers from coughs and colds in the winter, then echinacea, marshmallow, or mullein may be a good place to start.

Tips to Get You Started on Filling Up Your Herbal Medicine Cabinet

If you plan to grow your own herbs, try to plan your garden so that it is easy for you to access, and so that each plant will receive the ideal amount of sunlight that it needs. Some plants prefer to have as much sun as possible, and some plants prefer to have quite a bit of time in the shade. Do your research so that you know the soil conditions, sunlight requirements, and watering requirements that your herbs will require to make them happy and growing well year after year.

If you plan to forage for your herbs, try to find a few different areas to harvest the herbs from, and make sure that the areas that you use are not likely to be affected by pesticides or pollution. When foraging, make sure not to take more than 30% of the crop that is available. Some plants must be left in order to ensure that they will continue to grow as they provide a food source for many animals in wild areas. Again, it is important to do your research to make sure that you are harvesting the correct herbs, and not harvesting plants that may potentially be dangerous.

Make sure that you have an appropriate space to dry your herbs since most preparations require herbs that are fully dried. A basement or a cupboard works well as long as the herbs can be allowed to hang for several months without being disturbed. They should not be kept outside or in a bathroom, or anywhere else that may have high humidity

Collect jars and bottles with lids, pumps, droppers, in which to store your herbal preparations.

Chapter 7 : Herbal Medication First Aid Kit

Building a first aid kit is a great way to get to know about some useful herbs, and it is a good idea to have these simple preparations with you when you go out or when you travel so that you can be prepared for any situation that may arise without relying on over-the-counter medical preparations. Below are listed some of the more common things that can happen when out and about, and some simple herbal preparations that you can make ahead of time to take with you.

Cuts and Scrapes

Cuts and scrapes happen easily, so having a healing salve on hand that is safe to use on adults and kids is a great idea. When making this salve, divide it between a large pot for keeping at home and a smaller pot or a twist-up lip balm container to carry with you.

Calendula and Plantain Salve

The first step is to make two herbal oils, one from calendula petals and one from plantain leaves. Any base oil can be used for these, but either Sweet Almond or Olive oils would be a good choice because of their stable shelf lives and anti-inflammatory properties.

Once the oils are made, mix ½ cup each of the calendula and plantain oils with ¼ cup of beeswax to make the salve. When carrying a beeswax salve with you, keep in mind that it has the potential to melt when exposed to high temperatures. When possible, keep this salve on ice until needed.

Burns

Whether from a fire, from a hot element, or from the sun, burns can happen any time and need quick treatment. A salve made from calendula and aloe vera is a great one to have on hand to soothe minor burns.

Aloe and Calendula Salve

Make an aloe salve by combining equal parts of the gel from an aloe leaf and olive oil. Prepare a salve with calendula oil and beeswax, and then take it off the heat and mix the aloe salve in before placing it into a pot.

Upset Stomach

There are many things that can cause an upset stomach when traveling, from the food to illness to anxiety from the travel itself. Teas can easily be made ahead of time and stored in either zip-top bags or small jars or in empty tea bags available commercially.

Marshmallow and Peppermint Tea

Mix equal amounts of dried marshmallow root and dried peppermint leaves and then add one tablespoon of the mixture into each tea bag for use while traveling.

Muscle Aches

Calendula, Chickweed, and Elderflower Oil

In a glass jar, place a mixture of calendula petals, chickweed flowers and petals, and elderflowers. Fill the jar with jojoba oil, which works well for anti-inflammatory purposes. Leave the jar for at least three weeks, and then strain, and then the oil can either be stored in a tight-fitting jar in your first aid kit or can be made into a salve for easy transportation.

Sore throat, Cough, Colds, Upper Respiratory Tract Infections

For a sore throat or a cough, a lozenge that will coat the throat with healing medicine is just the trick. These lozenges are easy to make and easy to carry around when needed. Take care that they do not get wet. Store them in an empty tin or jar.

Marshmallow, Burdock, and Peppermint Lozenges

Place one tablespoon of dried marshmallow root in a bowl with ¼ cup of water overnight. To the resultant gel, add two tablespoons of honey and ½ cup of powdered marshmallow root. Make a decoction of burdock root with ½ cup water and two tablespoons of dried burdock root simmered for 20 minutes. Remove this from the heat and add three tablespoons of dried peppermint leaf. Steep for 15 minutes and then add this to the bowl with the marshmallow root. Stir all together to make a dough and roll it out to about ½ inch thick. More powdered marshmallow root or water can be added to adjust the dough and make it wetter or drier. Cut the rolled dough into individual lozenges and lay them out on a cookie sheet to dry. These can be dried using a dehydrator, or they can be placed in an oven on the lowest setting for one to two hours.

Anxiety, Sleep, Stress

Traveling may be stressful for some, and it may also be difficult to get a good sleep while traveling. For travel-related anxiety, a pill from oats and valerian can help to settle nerves and ensure a good night's sleep.

Valerian and Oatstraw Pills

Mix one cup of dried and powdered oatstraw with one cup of dried and powdered valerian. Mix well and place into gelatin capsules.

Allergic Reactions or Itchy Skin

As long as there is not a severe allergic reaction such as breathing trouble, or a rash that spreads over the entire body, a mild allergic reaction on the skin may be calmed by applying a salve of dandelion and plantain.

Dandelion and Plantain Salve

Using dried plantain leaves and dried dandelion flowers, create an herbal oil. Using grapeseed oil as the base is a good idea since it is less likely to contribute to an allergic reaction. The two oils can be made separately or may be infused in the same jar. Once the oil is ready, mix with beeswax as outlined above to make a soothing and calming salve for irritated skin.

www.ingramcontent.com/pod-product-compliance
Lightning Source LLC
Chambersburg PA
CBHW070704250726
48662CB00001B/242